UPDATED EDITION

BIG FAT LIES

THE TRUTH ABOUT
YOUR WEIGHT
AND
YOUR HEALTH

GLENN A. GAESSER, PH.D.

gürze books

Big Fat Lies
The Truth about Your Weight and Your Health
Updated Edition

©2002 by Glenn A. Gaesser, Ph.D.

Gürze Books
PO Box 2238
Carlsbad, CA 92018
(800) 756-7533
www.gurze.com

Cover design by Abacus Graphics, Oceanside, CA.

This is a first trade paperback, updated edition of a hardcover book originally published by Ballantine Books in 1996. In this 2002 edition, the author has updated and revised the entire text.

Grateful acknowledgment is made to the following for permission to reprint previously published material: *Annual Reviews Inc.*: Excerpt from "The Problem of Obesity" by Faith Fitzgerald, *Annual Review of Medicine*, Volume 32, © 1981 by Annual Reviews Inc. *Carol Mann Agency*: Excerpt from *Never Too Thin: Why Women Are at War with Their Bodies* by Roberta Pollack Seid, Prentice Hall Press. © 1989 by Roberta Pollack Seid. *Metropolitan Life Insurance Company*: Excerpt from *Statistical Bulletin* reprinted courtesy of Metropolitan Life Insurance Company. *The New England Journal of Medicine*: Excerpt from "News about Obesity" by Paul Ernsberger and Paul Haskew, Volume 315, No. 2, July 10, 1986, pages 130-131. © 1991 Massachusetts Medical Society.

Library of Congress Catalog Number: 2002105583
ISBN 0-936077-42-5

The authors and publishers of this book intend for this publication to provide accurate information. It is sold with the understanding that it is meant to complement, not substitute for, professional, medical, and/or psychological services.

3 5 7 9 0 8 6 4 2

For my mother, Mary—
thin and hypertensive,
she may well have benefited
from a few extra pounds.

CONTENTS

ACKNOWLEDGMENTS

On the afternoon of June 17, 1972, on the campus of the University of California, Berkeley, a student delivered a speech to the graduating class of the department of physical education. It seemed appropriate that the speech focused on the role of exercise in preventive medicine, and specifically on what the graduates might contribute to society in this regard. In the speech the student proclaimed "obesity is a disease" and warned of its perils in much the same manner as a panel of scientists would do some thirteen years later at an NIH-sponsored conference in Bethesda, Maryland. I was that student; little did I know then that I would one day write *BIG FAT LIES: The Truth About Your Weight and Your Health.*

For me, the turnabout on the obesity/health issue stemmed from two things. For one, the health and vigor of many heavier-than-average men and women I encountered over the years—some in the laboratory, some in my clinical experience—seemed to defy the dire warnings I had conveyed in my graduation speech. To those who provided living proof of this book's thesis, and gave me their time and told me their stories, I am deeply indebted. However, it wasn't until I began to explore the scientific literature on the subject—as preparation for classes I taught at UCLA in the 1980s and now teach at the University of Virginia—that I realized that there was a story to tell. The end result of my explorations is this book.

Since I am not the first to challenge the mainstream view on obesity and health, I must acknowledge the works of others, for they profoundly shaped my (re)thinking on the matter. Foremost among these individuals are Ancel Keys and Reubin Andres, pioneers who were way ahead of their time; if only we had listened. Hilde Bruch (*The Importance of Overweight*, in 1957), William Bennett and Joel Gurin (*The Dieter's Dilemma: Eating Less and Weighing More*, in 1982), Janet Polivy and C. Peter Herman (*Breaking the Diet Habit: The Natural Weight Alternative*, in 1983), Hillel Schwartz (*Never Satisfied: A Cultural History of Diets, Fantasies, and Fat*, in 1986), Paul Ernsberger and Paul Haskew (*Rethinking Obesity: An Alternative View of its Health Implications*, in 1987), and Roberta Pollack

Seid (*Never Too Thin: Why Women Are at War with Their Bodies*, in 1989), also opened my eyes; their voices, too, resonate in this book.

Credit for this book must also go to my teachers, especially George Brooks, Larry Rarick, and Brian Whipp, who showed me the way of science and taught me to, above all, keep an open mind; Leonard Marascuilo, who taught me that statistics is more about common sense than about numbers; and to Bob Card, who made me realize that education is so much more than schooling.

A very special thanks to Jim Barnard and Steven Blair for sharing their time and insights, and for providing me with a steady stream of scientific evidence to help build the foundation upon which this book is based.

I thank Carol Otis, John Kral, Priscilla Clarkson, and Tim White for their careful read of the original version of the manuscript and suggestions for edits. Some of their suggestions were incorporated, and some were not. If you disagree with anything in this book, however, do not blame them—I take full responsibility for presentation of the material in this book.

For their insight, inspiration, encouragement, and unwavering support of the "health at every size" paradigm, special thanks to Francie Berg, Debby Burgard, Paul Ernsberger, Cheri Erdman, Dayle Hayes, Joanne Ikeda, Nancy King, Karin Kratina, Pat Lyons, Lynn McAfee, and Jon Robison.

I acknowledge my agent, Lynn Seligman, who made it possible for me to get my proposal in the right hands, and I thank Jonathan Coleman for recommending her.

The finished product, of course, would not be what it is without the help of wonderful editors. My wife, Patricia, read every word of every draft of the first edition more times than she cares to remember. I believe that her editorial comments had a lot to do with the decision of Ginny Faber, my editor at Ballantine, to give a first-time author a chance. To Ginny, I say "thank you"—for giving me that chance, and for believing that this book has an important message. I also owe a great deal to Beth Rashbaum, who just has to be the best text editor a writer could ever want.

I also want to thank Leigh Cohn of Gürze Books for providing me the opportunity to publish this updated version of *BIG FAT LIES,* and Elaine Moore for her wonderful editing skills.

The research and writing of this book took the better part of five years. It made for a lot of late nights and working weekends. Through it all, my family was tremendously supportive. To Patricia and my terrific children, Mike, Lindsay, and Brandon, thanks for your patience and understanding—you make it all worthwhile.

Finally, my deepest thanks to my parents, Mary and Richard, for making it all possible.

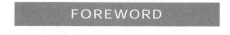

by Steven N. Blair, PED

Director of Research, The Cooper Institute for Aerobics Research; Senior Scientific Editor, Surgeon General's Report on Physical Activity and Health

Millions of Americans, most of them women, step on the bathroom scale each morning and let it dictate the kind of day they will have. If their weight is down a pound or two, it will be a good day; if it's up a pound, the day is already off to a bad start. So it goes in a "thin is in" culture that has brainwashed us to believe that the numbers on the bathroom scale tell us something meaningful about our worth. Americans spend tens of billions of dollars each year in an effort to lose weight, trying—mostly in vain—to conform to the cultural standard of the "ideal" or "desirable" body shape, which, at least for women, has become progressively thinner over the past few decades. Unfortunately, the average American woman (and man, for that matter) is heavier now than ever before, which means that a good many of us are having quite a few "bad scale days."

While these "bad scale days" are damaging to our self-esteem and our emotional well-being, much of what is written about the ever-widening gap between what we actually weigh and what we are told we should weigh focuses on health. It is at this issue—the alleged health hazard of being overweight—that *BIG FAT LIES: The Truth about Your Weight and Your Health*, takes aim. And it is right on target. One of the most firmly held and widely accepted views in the weight loss industry and in medical circles is that overweight *itself* constitutes a major health crisis, and that weight loss in overweight individuals results in improved health and better chances for avoiding premature death.

Herein lies the paradox. It is absolutely clear that elevated blood pressure and cholesterol can cause heart attacks and other health problems. It is also well-established that weight loss, even in those only mildly overweight, will lower blood pressure and cholesterol. Therefore, it seems logical to conclude that weight loss in overweight individuals will reduce their risk of heart attack, stroke, diabetes, perhaps some types of cancer, and of death from these diseases. It should follow that if a large population of overweight individuals have their weight measured over time, those who lose weight would be less likely to suffer premature death from cardiovascular diseases and other causes than those who do not lose weight. Furthermore, we might expect that when overweight individuals gain even more weight, they are more likely to die prematurely than overweight persons who do not. Yet these expectations, as Dr. Gaesser's book makes strikingly clear, are *not* well-supported by existing studies.

In one study that I helped direct, we examined more than 12,000 men who were at high risk for heart disease. We measured their body weights one or more times per year for a period of six to seven years, then kept track of mortality statistics on these men for nearly four years. Contrary to conventional wisdom, weight loss did not lower the death rates of these high-risk men. In fact, compared to men whose weights remained reasonably stable over the six to seven years (even if those weights were *above* the recommended range), men who lost weight actually had a *greater* risk of dying during the nearly four years of follow-up. Although this was most pronounced in the thinnest men, we observed the same thing in men who were moderately overweight. To say the least, these findings were unexpected. These high-risk men are exactly the individuals who should benefit from weight loss, but the data did not support this hypothesis.

One study of a very large population of overweight, nonsmoking women showed some benefit in terms of reduced mortality for women who intentionally lost weight, but this was true only for those women with preexisting health problems (such as high blood pressure or a history of heart trouble). The overweight women in this study who had no health problems received no benefit from losing weight. An additional finding that defied conventional wisdom was that weight *gain* did not pose any threat to the longevity prospects for these overweight women.

I mention these two studies to highlight the inconsistency, unexpected findings, and paradoxical information that exist in the scientific literature on weight loss. They are by no means the rare exceptions. Instead, they typify a preponderance of scientific information that tells us we need to seriously rethink the purported link between body weight and health, the actual meaning of "overweight," and the virtually unquestioned assumption that weight loss is a desirable goal for the more than one-half of U.S. adults who are currently classified as "overweight." Conventional wisdom on body weight, weight loss, and health can, and should, be questioned.

Dr. Gaesser's provocative examination of the science on this topic, and his straightforward consideration of difficult issues and questions make this book a "must read" for all those interested in understanding the relationship of body weight to health as well as the potential repercussions of endless attempts to lose weight. His honest presentation of a vast number of studies on various aspects of body weight and health will challenge—and most likely reshape—your thinking on these issues.

Dr. Gaesser encourages us to pursue a healthy lifestyle as the most important barometer of fitness. His Twenty/Twenty Program for Metabolic Fitness calls for an average of 20 minutes of physical activity per day and a target goal for fat consumption of an average of 20 percent of your total calories. Most fitness programs place far too much emphasis on body weight. Many weight control programs specify an ideal body weight, and set a definite weight loss goal. This is a silly approach.

Scientists can calculate the average weight-for-height that is associated with the lowest mortality rate in a given population, but this does not mean, as it is frequently interpreted, that this is an ideal weight for all persons of a given height. The approach of setting a specific target weight concentrates our attention on the scale rather than on our lifestyles. With Dr. Gaesser's program, you can ignore the height-weight tables, toss your bathroom scale, and say good-bye forever to those "bad scale days."

Thin people do not have a monopoly on health and fitness. Fit and healthy bodies come in all shapes and sizes—as my research at the Cooper Institute for Aerobics Research has shown. By tracking the health status of thousands of women and men who have had fitness tests and medical exams at the Institute over the past thirty years or so, it has become abundantly clear to me that in terms of health and longevity, your fitness level is far more important than your weight. If the height-weight charts say you are 5 pounds too heavy, or even 50 or more pounds too heavy, it is of little consequence healthwise—*as long as you are physically fit*. On the other hand, if you are a couch potato, being thin provides absolutely no assurance of good health, and does nothing to increase your chances of living a long life. A "good scale day" may do wonders for your vanity, but it tells you little about your health.

The Twenty/Twenty program is a great way to get those of us who don't do any regular physical activity—which, by the way, is as many as 40 to 50 million American adults—on our way to a healthier lifestyle. It is remarkably flexible, and thus doable, in contrast to the overly prescriptive and structured programs often recommended to the public. As my research has shown, the greatest reductions in premature death rates are achieved by totally unfit people who become just moderately fit. Similarly, Dr. Gaesser found that the men and women who stand to gain the most from his program are those who go from nothing to something, such as the 20 minutes-per-day target he recommends. Of course, doing a bit more—either more minutes at the moderate-intensity level that Dr. Gaesser advocates for starters, or by staying at the 20 minutes-per-day minimum and gradually increasing the intensity—will likely benefit you even more. The bottom line is still quite simple: Try to be more active.

Some may find that the target of 20 percent of total calories from fat a bit difficult to achieve, especially considering that the average American now consumes close to 35 percent of his or her daily calories from fat. But again, it's not a rigid goal. Like the recommendation for physical activity, every little bit helps. There is no doubt in my mind that if sedentary individuals who eat the typical American diet would follow Dr. Gaesser's Twenty/Twenty Program for Metabolic Fitness, they would significantly improve their prospects for a long and healthy life.

BIG FAT LIES

Do you believe that your weight should be within the range recommended by one of the various height-weight tables that are always appearing in books, magazines, and health-profession handouts? That being overweight is unhealthy? That weight loss improves health?

Have you ever been told by your doctor to lose weight? Are you currently dieting or contemplating going on a diet? Have diets failed you or made you feel like a failure? Do you feel people look down on you because of your weight? If the answer to any of these questions is "yes," then this book is for you.

Anything but a "yes" answer to the first three questions might seem heretical. After all, nearly every medical and health organization in the United States has taken the position that obesity is a major health hazard. We are told that most of us are too fat, and that this is very bad. Virtually all health and fitness professionals routinely point to one or another of the height-weight tables or relatively new body mass index charts and recommend that their "overweight" patients lose enough weight to fall within the designated ranges. No wonder most of us believe that thinner is better, obesity is a disease, weight loss invariably improves health, and a "fat" person cannot, by definition, be "fit," since body fat is intrinsically bad.

Those beliefs are so firmly entrenched in our fat-phobic mind-set that they are seldom questioned, but they should be. The idea that a given body weight, or a percentage of body fat, is a meaningful indicator of health, fitness, or prospects for longevity is one of our most firmly-held beliefs, and one of our most dubious propositions. There is a large and ever-growing body of scientific evidence, most of it still confined to professional journals, showing that fat may not be so bad and thin may not be so good. This is not to say that obesity is entirely benign or that body weight is unimportant to health. It's just that when you scrutinize all the relevant data it becomes apparent that the health risks of obesity, as well as the purported health benefits of weight loss, have been greatly exaggerated. Furthermore, the risks associated with weight loss have been underestimated.

In most instances, "excess" body fat might be more aptly considered a symptom, not a direct cause, of disease. It could also be called an "imprecise marker for an imprudent lifestyle," as two researchers argued some years ago in the *New England Journal of Medicine*. The health risks associated with obesity are much the same as those associated with a sedentary lifestyle and poor diet (which also contribute to obesity). The fact that some of the most common health problems associated with obesity, such as high blood pressure, glucose intolerance, and blood lipid disorders, can be ameliorated independently of weight loss supports this viewpoint.

This observation, however, is but one of many evidence-based challenges to the conventional wisdom on body weight and health. Consider the following:

- State-of-the-art techniques used to assess the degree to which fat deposits clog arteries—the chief, underlying cause of cardiovascular disease—in most instances show that there is no connection between fat-clogged arteries and obesity. Fat *in* the arteries and fat *on* the body are different and not necessarily related.

- Body fat can actually be beneficial, depending on its location. Thigh and hip fat, for example, have been reported to be associated with lower risk of cardiovascular disease and possibly type 2 diabetes, especially in women.

- Men and women medically classified as "overweight" or "obese" who exercise regularly and are physically fit, yet remain above the ranges recommended by the height-weight tables or body mass index charts, have lower all-cause death rates than thin men and women who do not exercise and are unfit.

- Men and women medically classified as "overweight" or "obese" have lower risks for lung cancer (in both smokers and non-smokers) and osteoporosis than men and women who are either thin or of average weight.

- Weight loss does not necessarily improve health or lengthen life. Dieters, especially yo-yo dieters, who make up the vast majority of dieters in this country and whose weights fluctuate considerably throughout their adult lives, have a risk for cardio-vascular disease and type 2 diabetes (the most common kind) that is up to twice that of "overweight" people who remain fat. Most studies of the impact of weight loss on mortality rates show the "lose weight, live longer" axiom to be a myth.

- The "thinner is better" studies frequently cited by health professionals are far outnumbered by studies showing that— aside from the very extremes—body weight is fairly unrelated to health status and death rates or that weights above those recommended by the height-weight tables are actually better for health and longevity.

Our belief that "thinner is better" often has nothing to do with health, even when it is a member of the health establishment itself who is promoting it. One of the most poignant examples of this phenom-enon was a woman I knew who considered herself a terrible "failure" because of her weight. Years before, Betty had joined a health club because, at five feet seven inches tall, 137 pounds, and 28 percent body fat, she had decided she was overweight. Soon she was working out at a health club with a personal trainer, who not only didn't discourage her from trying to pursue some impossible ideal, but chastised her one day for having gained one pound in the preceding month. The fact that during the time she had been working out with him she had lowered her blood pressure substantially and maintained her already excellent cholesterol levels didn't sway him a bit. He urged her to work all the harder to "reverse this serious trend in body weight."

Soon afterward, Betty dropped out of the health club. Ashamed of her "failure" and discouraged by her inability to lose weight, she figured "Why bother to exercise?" and turned to the standard approach to weight loss: dieting. She dieted off and on for years, with the result that by her mid-fifties, she weighed 170 pounds and had a body fat composition of just over 40 percent. I met her at that point because she joined the Cardiovascular Health and Fitness Program at the University of Virginia, her single "fitness" goal being to return to the dress size she had been in high school. Though she did very well on the program, once again lowering her blood pressure as well as increasing her aerobic capacity and endurance, she didn't lose much weight; since she hadn't gotten anywhere near her goal, she eventually dropped out of our program, too. She is the typical fitness dropout, the typical diet "failure."

But she is only a dropout and a failure because her goal had been wrongly defined. When the combined forces of the medical establishment, the life insurance industry, and the fashion world dictate weight standards, as has happened for at least the past 50 years or so, the real goals of the changes most of us need to make in nutrition and exercise habits—improved health and longevity—get lost. And the real indicators of improved health and longevity, which have little to do with weight, get obscured.

Dieting: The False Way to Fitness and to Health

One of the first inklings that weight might not be a key factor in health came to me a number of years ago via a student. As part of one of my classes in exercise physiology, I asked the students to agree to be weighed, measured for body fat, and given an exercise stress test. At five feet ten inches tall, Mike weighed 230 pounds and had 32 percent body fat—by medical standards obese. However, he exercised regularly and, as I discovered when he took the stress test, had an impressive oxygen uptake capacity. In fact, he outperformed more than 95 percent of his peers, whom he also outweighed. Seventy-four pounds of body fat notwithstanding, Mike had an aerobic fitness level that was, by anyone's standards, superb. No fitness expert in America would have classified a man with that much body fat as fit, however, because "fat" has been defined as the opposite of "fit." The truth is that weight has little, if anything, to do with either fitness or health. But that's not the story that has been drummed into us over the years.

Americans have been deceived. The overwhelming evidence against this deception has largely been ignored, not just by those with a stake in the more than $30 billion a year weight-loss industry, which was founded on our belief that fat is unhealthy, but by a scientific community similarly biased against fat and mired in conservatism and inertia. The results of this deception are very serious indeed—not just in wasted money, but in damage to health and even loss of life. Conservative estimates say that 90 percent of dieters ultimately regain the pounds they lose. (Many of them eventually go on another diet as part of an endless cycle of weight lost and regained.) In Chapter 7, I will describe the results of many studies that suggest that the consequences of perpetual dieting and constant weight fluctuation may ultimately be fatal. However, few of the vast numbers of repeat dieters are aware of the risks they are running.

Let's face it: Millions of heavier-than-average men and women have been victimized, and their health jeopardized, by the attack on what a distinguished physician once described as one of our body's "most peaceful, useful, and law-abiding...tissues."

Take Wanda, for example. Wanda went on her first diet when she was fifteen years old, because at five feet six inches tall and 145 pounds, she thought she was fat. By age forty-two she had gone through fifty-some diets and weighed over 240 pounds. She can't remember how many times she was told, "You really should do something about your weight." And she always did—by dieting. That, alas, was unfortunate because, contrary to what we are led to believe, dieting almost always promotes the very thing it is supposed to cure: obesity. Countless studies show that yo-yo dieting, or what one expert called the "rhythm method of girth control," is the kind of dieting that most people do, and that it usually culminates not just in weight regained but also in additional weight being put on. Wanda, like Betty and millions of others, has learned this the hard way.

Wanda's plight represents the essence of this book. I will provide a wealth of scientific data to debunk the dogma that our body fat is killing us and that dieting is a panacea. Body fat is not intrinsically unhealthy. Dieting, on the other hand, can be. Chances are, dieting is never going to make us either healthier or better looking (at least not for long). One reason for this is that, contrary to the calorie equation that is presented to us in every diet book, whereby 3,500 calories equal one pound of body fat, and if you eat 3,500 calories fewer per week, you will lose one pound, the human body is not infinitely malleable. It's not a simple input and output machine but a complex, living organism. Thus you cannot redesign your body via a simple calorie-consumption and burn-off equation. All kinds of factors, ranging from genes to body chemistry to the irreversibility of fat-cell increases, render such an equation meaningless. The proof of this lies in the fact that, despite decades of increasingly intense efforts at weight loss through dieting, the average American is about 15 pounds heavier today than a mere 20 years ago.

However, what I referred to above as Wanda's plight is only half of her story; the other half is also part of the essence of this book. At sixty-four, Wanda decided to make physical activity a part of her life. She also has moved from ceaseless dieting to an acceptance of her weight, which she estimates to be something over 200 pounds. She doesn't know exactly what it is because she doesn't care. "What matters is my health," she says. "I try to exercise regularly, cut out fatty foods, and focus only on things I can do something about—like my blood sugar and choles-terol levels, and blood pressure. I'm sorry that I wasted nearly fifty years of my life trying to do something about what others told me I should do something about."

Metabolic Fitness: The New Approach to Health and Longevity

Wanda's focus on blood pressure, blood sugar, and blood cholesterol levels is in response to a different concept of fitness, which only now is beginning to be recognized. Fitness is not integrally related to weight, nor should it be limited to measures of cardiorespiratory capacity and endurance, which have for decades dominated our notion of fitness and turned millions of people into pulse-takers. The measurements in which Wanda is interested constitute the basic parameters of a new definition of fitness, which I call "metabolic fitness." They are what I was talking about above when I referred to the "real indicators of improved health and longevity." Achieving metabolic fitness is probably the most important thing you can do for your physical health, and is thus the underlying theme of this entire book, as well as the explicit goal of the final three chapters. The physical activity and nutrition guidelines presented in those chapters, which constitute what I call the Twenty/Twenty Program for Metabolic Fitness, will help you achieve that goal, regardless of whether you lose weight.

Weight loss, however, remains a major health goal of the medical establishment, even when all the "overweight" person's vital statistics indicate good health. Consider Tess, for example, who at forty-eight years of age, five feet five inches tall and 160 pounds, is considered overweight by the relatively new body mass index criteria (which is defined and discussed in chapter 2). Tess eats a low-fat, high-fiber diet, exercises regularly, and has normal blood pressure; her blood cholesterol and blood sugar levels fall well within healthy ranges. Tess is an active, vibrant, energetic person who feels good almost all the time—except when she has to go for a medical checkup. She dreads seeing her doctor, because he always harangues her about her weight. Switching doctors doesn't help, either. The message is always the same: Lose weight. She's tried, but never with any lasting success. She now states emphatically that "I can't lose weight, and I'm not going to try anymore." Her constant efforts to lose, which always ended in defeat, made her feel "less of a person every day." Now she feels comfortable with herself, accepting that she is probably at her "natural" body weight—the weight her now middle-aged body *prefers.* Each person's natural weight is unique to him or her and will not be found on any height-weight table. Like Tess, who may have inadvertently upped her "natural" weight by years of dieting or as a result of periods of very sedentary living and/or overeating, some people have relatively heavy weights.

Others, like my friend Charlotte, seem naturally to fall at the lighter end of the weight continuum. Charlotte is five feet five inches tall, weighs 128 pounds, has excellent blood pressure readings and a terrific blood fat profile (which assesses cholesterol and triglyceride levels in the blood). Is her doctor pleased? No. For whatever reason, perhaps because she is employing some personal standard that is even stricter than those in the height-weight tables, the doctor has told Charlotte that she is "mildly overweight." But if Charlotte were to lose weight, what purpose would it serve? Certainly not to improve her vital signs, which are all excellent. Actually a while ago Charlotte did have a slightly elevated cholesterol level. At 220 mg/dl (milligrams of cholesterol per deciliter of blood), she was 20 milligrams above the upper limit recommended as healthy by the National Cholesterol Education Program. She was not, however, overweight, by any standard. By cutting out most of the high-fat dairy products she'd been eating, she reduced her cholesterol to a very desirably low 170 mg/dl in almost no time. Because she had cut her fat intake considerably, she also eventually lost a couple of pounds, but the cholesterol level plummeted long before the weight dropped—proving, as I've seen time and again and as numerous studies confirm, that weight has nothing to do with cholesterol levels. And this underscores another major theme of my book: It's primarily the fat (particularly saturated fat) in the diet, not on the body, that poses the real threat to health.

Health at Every Size

If we can accept the fact that healthy bodies come in many shapes and sizes and begin to view exercise and diet as more than just means to an end (weight loss), then the public health message becomes much more clear: People should be physically active, eat healthy foods, and not obsess about the numbers on the scale. The "health at every size" paradigm allows for a compassionate and open-minded view of body weight and may have a positive impact on public health. Millions of Americans stigmatized as "too fat" need to be reassured that the roads to good health are wide enough for everyone.

This book was written in an effort to provide that reassurance, and with the hope of discrediting the myths that obesity is a "killer disease," that weight loss is inherently good, that thinner is necessarily healthier, and that the height-weight tables measure something meaningful. Given that these myths have proved Teflon-like in their ability to repel facts in the past, I know that even the myriad of data I will be hurling against them may not do the job immediately. But I also know that if you subject it to sufficient abrasion for long enough, even Teflon eventually wears away.

PART

1

THE CRUSADE AGAINST OBESITY

CHAPTER 1

Weight:
An Unhealthy Obsession

It is clear from reading magazines or watching television that public derision and condemnation of fat people is one of the few remaining sanctioned social prejudices in this nation freely allowed against any group based solely on appearance.

—Faith Fitzgerald, M.D. "The Problem of Obesity,"
Annual Review of Medicine, 1981

Dr. Fitzgerald's assertion is, technically speaking, only 98 percent correct. One state in the Union does not sanction the prejudice against fat people. The Elliott-Larsen Civil Rights Act, which was approved by the governor of Michigan in 1977 and has remained on the books ever since, prohibits discrimination on the basis of weight. This one unique act of legislation notwithstanding, it is fair to say that Dr. Fitzgerald's statement accurately describes the extremely negative view of our society toward all those who happen to fall on the "heavy" end of the bell-shaped curve describing the weight ranges for any given height.

Fat people are routinely described as "ugly," "disgusting," "sloppy," and "gross," and characterized as "weak-willed," "self-indulgent," "lacking in self-respect," "emotionally disturbed," and possibly "sick." Occasionally, the descriptions even veer into moral judgments, as we denounce the fat person for failure to maintain his health for the sake of his family by saying "If he doesn't care enough to lose weight for his own good, he could at least think about *them*," or chide him for embarrassing his children in front of their friends. Is it any wonder, then, that heavy people can be made to feel, as some of the fat people I have encountered over the years put it, "less of a person every day"? If the attitudes of the society at large are not damning enough, surveys indicate that up to 88 percent of our health care professionals share some or all of these feelings. Indeed the medical establishment has been largely responsible for our anti-fat crusade, giving it the imprimatur of science and thereby legitimizing it. In 1994, when former surgeon general C. Everett Koop initiated his "Shape Up America" campaign, he asserted that obesity is responsible for almost a thousand deaths a day in the United States.

Medical, moral, and esthetic condemnation of fat is now so pervasive in the United States that it ranks as a distinctive cultural trait. Fat phobia has become epidemic. We want fat-free bodies and the fat-free foods we think will help us to attain them. However, only the very few will ever achieve the cultural ideal—and many of the "successes" only at serious risk to their health. The unattainability of the goal we have set for ourselves explains why we have become so profoundly dissatisfied with our bodies. A 1994 *Prevention* magazine women's fitness survey indicated that more than 50 percent of women were either "not very" or "not at all" satisfied with their bodies, and that 90 percent said they needed to lose weight. Statistics among young people are even worse. Nearly 80 percent of the eighteen-year-old girls in one survey expressed dissatisfaction with their bodies. In addition, "getting fat" is cited by a considerable percentage of teenagers and young adults—mainly female— as being their greatest fear. In a poll of one thousand women between the ages of eighteen and twenty-five, which ran in the February 1994 issue of *Esquire*, 54 percent stated that they would rather be run over by a truck than be extremely fat. Two-thirds said they would rather be mean or stupid than fat.

What is most amazing about these figures is that of all the millions of men and women who feel so unhappy about their bodies, many are at a weight that is within the ranges currently recommended by the U.S. government. Our fear of fat, though, has at least as much to do with vanity as it does with health. While a significant number of dieters cite medical reasons for their desire to shed pounds, most of us are more concerned with improving our appearance in a society where only thin is in. Our self-image and our self-esteem suffer if we do not look like the models and movie stars who constitute our ideal. As a result we are now a population obsessed with losing weight, usually by dieting.

Diet Mania

Just how obsessive Americans have become about dieting is dramatically revealed by the results of two recent large-scale surveys conducted under the auspices of the U.S. government, both published in the *Journal of the American Medical Association*. By combining these survey results with data obtained from the 2000 U.S. census, roughly 25 million men are said to be dieting to lose weight at any given time, and 43 million women. About 21 million men are dieting to maintain weight, and a little more than 26 million women. In total, there are nearly 116 million adults dieting at any given time, representing about 55 percent of the total adult population. By contrast, a Louis Harris poll in 1964 indicated that only 15 percent of adults were dieting. Among adolescents, about 3 million girls and 1 million boys say they are "skipping meals" to lose weight. The total, then, stands at about 120 million Americans over the age of eleven trying to lose or maintain weight by one form or another of calorie deprivation.

For most dieters the obsession is cyclical in nature: the average dieter spends roughly six months of every year actively trying to lose weight—and, as is frequently the case, the other six months gaining most if not all, or more, of the weight back. For women in particular, the obsession can be almost ceaseless: In one survey, nearly one-third of the women between the ages of nineteen and thirty-nine admitted to dieting at least once a month, while 16 percent consider themselves perpetual dieters. Dieting as a way of life begins early. Eighty percent of the teenage girls in the United States have been on at least one diet. Dieting has even become common among children—mainly girls—in grade school. Is it any wonder that our young girls and women are experiencing an epidemic of anorexia and bulimia? Or that the same problems are beginning to afflict young men?

Americans have become easy marks for anyone trying to sell weight loss, by *any* means. The 120 million people who are trying to lose or maintain weight via reduced calorie intake have turned dieting into a $30-billion-plus industry (with some estimates much higher than that). We participate by the millions in such weight-loss programs as Weight Watchers, Jenny Craig, and TOPS (Take Off Pounds Sensibly), paying fees to attend their meetings and, in some cases, buying their packaged food products as well. But this kind of dieting tells only part of the story of our obsession. We also buy countless alleged "slimming" potions, prescription diet medications (anorectics), and other chemical cocktails. We are suckers for aversion therapy, hypnosis, and behavior-modification techniques designed to reduce our intake of food. As a last ditch, some of us have even had our stomachs stapled, our intestines bypassed, and our jaws wired shut. Of course, many of these drastic surgical procedures are performed for reasons said to be related to health. Nonetheless it's for aesthetic reasons that most of us yearn to be "fat-free," which is why the number-one cosmetic surgical technique now performed in the United States is liposuction. The American Society for Aesthetic Plastic Surgery reported 385,390 liposuction procedures performed in 2001 (more than breast augmentation—216,754—and face lift—117,034—combined). This represents an increase of 118 percent since 1997. Liposuction is now one of the most commonly performed surgical procedures of *any* type in the United States.

With roughly 40 percent of the entire U.S. population dieting at any one time, the amount of weight lost could be expected to be quite impressive. It is. By my reckoning, based on the Centers for Disease Control and Prevention (CDC) data, Americans lose roughly one billion pounds per year. Unfortunately, by another reckoning, the collective total weight gain is about one billion pounds per year—and then some. At any given time some are on their way down, others on their way back up. The weight-loss arena is like the stock market in this respect, but the generally positive trend of the stock market over time does not find a counterpart in the diet game. Year after year the weight gainers seem to outnumber the weight losers; in the end, practically everybody becomes a gainer. The average American is fatter now than at any other time in history. Between 1960 and 1980 the average weights of American men and women increased by only a few pounds. By 1991 the average adult weighed almost eight pounds more than U.S. adults did just a decade earlier. The sharp upward trend in weight gain during the 1980s appears not to have been a one-time anomaly. The results of eight annual surveys conducted by the U.S. Centers for Disease Control and Prevention in the 1990s indicated that the average U.S. adult was about seven pounds heavier in 1998 as compared to 1991. Year-by-year analyses revealed a virtually perfect linear increase of about one pound per year during the seven-year period. (A recent study published in the *New England Journal of Medicine* suggests that this may be due almost entirely to holiday weight gain.) All told, average U.S. adult weights have increased by roughly 15 pounds in the past 20 years. The trend is no different for our young citizens. Among children between the ages of six and eleven, the incidence of obesity has increased by more than 50 percent since 1963.

Why, with so many millions of Americans trying to lose weight, are so many of the same millions getting fatter? Basically there are three interrelated reasons. One, the average American is less physically active than at any other time in our history, and despite the passionate desire to lose weight, there is no evidence that we are about to reverse this trend. We have mistakenly opted to fight the battle of the bulge by reducing our calorie intake instead of increasing our caloric expenditure via exercise. Only 10 to 20 percent of men and women trying to lose or maintain weight get in at least 150 minutes of physical activity per week—the minimum amount recommended by the U.S. surgeon general. Two, Americans now consume about fifteen to twenty pounds more fat each year than our ancestors did 100 years ago. Eating fat tends to make you fat. So, too, does dieting, which, ironically, is third on the list of reasons for Americans' expanding waistlines. A 1998 report on 19,478 male health professionals in the United States, for example, indicated that frequent dieting was related to subsequent weight gain. More recently, a 1999 report on 4,193 women and 3,536 men participating in the Finnish Twin Cohort Study revealed that dieters were several times more likely than non-dieters to experience major weight gain (more than 22 pounds) during a follow-up lasting 15 years. Data from one commercial weight-loss program indicated that 40 percent of participants gained back more weight than they had lost during the diet. Dieting, especially in a culture with a couch-potato lifestyle and plenty of high-fat fast foods instantly available to soothe the dieter's hunger cravings, promotes the very thing calorie restriction has been touted to cure: obesity.

Defending Our Fat Supplies

The first evidence of the fattening effect of dieting was provided more than half a century ago in a landmark study conducted by Dr. Ancel Keys. In 1944 Dr. Keys and his associates at the University of Minnesota designed a study that would enable them to investigate the physiological and psychological effects of severe, long-term energy (calorie) deprivation. Using as subjects thirty-two conscientious objectors who had been assigned to alternative service and were living in the university dormitories, they recorded the results of twenty-four weeks of living on a diet made up of slightly less than half the calories the men were accustomed to. As expected, all the men lost weight. Also as expected, they all put on weight when they were allowed to go off the diet, but they didn't just regain the weight they had lost; most gained several pounds more than that, all in the form of fat. Six of the men ended up with an average of nine and a half pounds more body fat than they had had before entering what became, in effect, the first controlled "yo-yo dieting" experiment.

The explanation for this phenomenon lies deep within our past and is part of our very genetic heritage. Back in the days of our hunter-gatherer ancestors, there was always uncertainty about when the next meal would be. Because there were often periods with little to eat, it was important that the human body be able to store what was consumed during the periods of plenty. Those whose bodies adapted by learning to store fat efficiently survived and reproduced, passing that ability on to their descendants; the others died out. The legacy of those feast and famine times is the "thrifty gene"—a genetic predisposition to hoard fat in preparation for the next famine. (This hoarding is accomplished via various biochemical adjustments and a strong tendency, in times of plenty, to have higher-than-normal levels of insulin in the blood, which greatly increases the storage capacity of each of the body's billions of fat cells.)

Naturally the bodies of the hunter-gatherer descendants do not distinguish between the recent phenomenon of self-induced starvation and the age-old problem of famine. Nature hasn't caught up with the fact that we are living in a time of plenty, calorie-wise. Thus, the human body, endowed with a remarkable capacity to make sure that once the missionary zeal with which most people begin their diets has given way to temptation, regains the lost pounds, usually with a vengeance. If this isn't discouraging enough news for the perpetual dieter, it's important to remember that in most cases nearly every ounce of the regained weight is in the form of fat, just as Dr. Keys's subjects proved.

From time immemorial and for reasons that are not entirely clear, gorging has been the typical response to periods of calorie deprivation, voluntary or otherwise. In the United States, gorging usually means bingeing on foods that were taboo during the diet—those laden with fat and sugar. Weight cycling, or "yo-yo dieting" as it is more commonly called, may really be better described as "fat cycling." A number of studies have shown that the inescapable consequence of repetitious cycles of weight loss and gain appears to be ever-greater accumulations of fat. With 120 million relatively sedentary dieters who live in a culture where fatty foods are abundant and popular, it's easy to understand why weight loss has become such an obsessive preoccupation, and why we have so many "failures" at it.

"Failure," of course, is a purely societal label. For the human body, the post-diet weight gain constitutes a success—success at defending what we call a "set-point weight." The set-point concept of body weight regulation will be explained in Chapter 5. Suffice it to say for the sake of the present discussion that the set point represents the weight that the body attempts to maintain, a weight that varies considerably from one person to another. Although a set-point weight may not remain "set" at one level over the course of an individual's adult lifetime, it does remain the same during the relatively short time frame of a typical diet. Dieting, then, is an attempt to defy the set point. Viewed in this manner, dieting is a thoroughly unnatural behavior. When a person's weight falls well below the set point, the body makes certain adjustments to thwart further assaults on its preferred weight. Ultimately, as the dismal data on dieting failures make clear, the body's set point is the winner in that battle.

Nature's victory is little comfort to the dieter. At war with our own bodies, we feel that *we* are the losers in the battle, *we* are the failures. The real winner, then, is the weight-loss industry. The body has given it the perfect fail-safe strategy to keep the customers stuck in a vicious cycle of weight loss and gain. But because we don't really understand what has gone wrong, we are vulnerable to blame-the-victim messages.

Diets don't fail, we are told, *dieters* do. The occasional high-profile dieter reinforces that message. In the 1980s, when Oprah Winfrey lost sixty-seven pounds on the Optifast program, sales for the company soared. When Oprah subsequently regained her weight, *she* was perceived as the failure, not the product or the philosophy behind the product. Of course, there's always the occasional success to inspire our continued hopes. After all, with 120 million dieters, even if 90 percent do regain the weight, that still leaves about 12 million people to offer up testimonials to whatever technique they used. All of us know one or two of these people, but they are very much the minority.

Our bad news is the weight-loss industry's boon, because it ensures a never-ending and ever-expanding supply of lucrative customers. The cost of shedding pounds can get very high. An analysis of one commercial weight-loss program estimated that it cost $180 per pound. The cost associated with prescription weight-loss drugs may be considerably higher. Although prices may vary, prescription weight-loss pills currently approved for use in the United States can be expected to cost at least $1,000 per year. Well-controlled studies show that pharmacotherapy rarely results in weight losses that are more than about 10 pounds greater than a comparison group receiving a placebo. Because the pills must be taken indefinitely in order to prevent weight regain (and even that is no guarantee that the pounds won't return), a young adult taking a weight-loss drug for life might shell out $40,000 for no more than a 10-pound "effect." That works out to at least $4,000 per pound!

The more than $30 billion a year Americans shelled out in the 1990s to slim down is now estimated to be close to $50 billion per year. Despite the less-than-stellar results achieved thus far, we seem bent on throwing good money after bad.

Other Costs
and Consequences of Dieting

In some ways wasted expenditure is the least of the costs the dieting mania has incurred. Twenty-five years ago eating disorders were very rare. The National Association of Anorexia Nervosa and Associated Disorders estimates that 8 million Americans, mostly young Caucasian women, currently suffer from either anorexia or bulimia, both of which can result in very serious medical problems, or from a more loosely defined grab-bag of other eating problems commonly referred to as binge-eating disorders. Although the cause of these various disorders is subject to much debate and is almost certainly a combination of many factors, the prevailing fat phobia of our culture is probably one of the significant contributors. We live in a society where women are conditioned to base much of their self-esteem on their success at maintaining a slim, girlish shape. Given that an irrational fear of fat is a common trait among those with eating disorders, it's not much of a leap to see a connection between their behavior and the cultural messages with which they are constantly being bombarded. Starvation diets are a hallmark of anorexia, and dieting is also believed by many of the leading experts in the field to be the major precipitator of the bingeing among bulimics.

As will be discussed in depth in later chapters, the health risks of dieting have been largely ignored. Dieting, particularly the yo-yo dieting that is very much the norm for millions of women, may increase the risk for a number of diseases, including cardiovascular disease, type 2 diabetes, osteoporosis, and certain cancers. Even mental function may be affected. One British study reported that 25 percent of girls ages 11 to 18 may be damaging their IQs as a result of dieting. In the deluge of facts and figures about the medical consequences of overweight, many of which are highly questionable, subject to multiple interpretations, or in outright error, this simple fact has gotten lost. If weight loss is embarked upon in the service of self-esteem, as is so often the case, imagine the psychological costs to those who are among the vast majority who fail at their goal. At a National Institutes of Health (NIH) conference on obesity it was acknowledged that "Obesity creates an enormous psychological burden. In terms of suffering, this burden may be the greatest adverse effect of obesity." Nonetheless, dieting to achieve some elusive ideal remains our national preoccupation. Low body weight is our measure of health, our symbol of self-worth.

Could it be that the health risks of overweight and obesity have been exaggerated? That body fat is less a health problem than our never-ending obsession with losing it? That what we commonly denounce as "overweight" and "obese" are dangerous only if they are the result of a diet too rich in junk foods and a daily regimen deficient in physical exercise? "Yes" to all of the above. For the millions of Americans trying to lose weight, whether they are doing it for the sake of their health or their appearance, a better understanding of the consequences of their actions is vital. Body fat is not lethal, but the effort to get rid of it can be.

Amazingly enough, despite our obsession with obesity, no acceptable health-oriented definition of obesity has ever been established. How much body fat is too much? How many pounds are too many? No one knows. Over the years, the attempt to come to grips with these questions has resulted in an endless series of height-weight tables, no two of which are the same; a contradictory and confusing overlap of such terms as *overweight*, *overfat*, and *obesity*; and multiple, often highly diverse ways of determining who is at risk. But our failure to agree on what constitutes obesity and when it becomes a health problem has not deterred us from agreeing on one simple, core belief: Obesity is bad. However, the truth is much more complex than that.

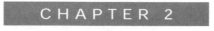

CHAPTER 2

How Obesity Got Such a Bad Name

This evil view of obesity has come from four places: the insurance industry, the medical moralizers (usually themselves thin), the drug industry and the docile, unquestioning nutritionists who are too often dupes of the faddists and hucksters.

—George V. Mann, M.D., "Obesity, the Nutritional Spook,"
American Journal of Public Health, 1971

A number of other culprits can be added to Dr. Mann's list, but two of them lead the pack: the fashion industry, which for most of this century has enthusiastically endorsed—and sometimes introduced—ever-thinner standards of appearance; and the fitness professionals, who have probably done more than any other group to make lean synonymous with healthy and fat with unhealthy. Collectively all these forces have conspired to portray obesity in the most disparaging terms possible.

Defining and Measuring Obesity

The negative attitude toward obesity even finds its way into medical, as well as standard, dictionaries, where the word is typically defined as "excessive bodily fat" or "excessive weight." The dictionaries do not generally distinguish *between* fat and weight (a distinction that has become fashionable only in the last few decades), nor do they define what "excessive" actually means. *Too much for what?* we might ask; but the answer is nowhere to be found.

Since dictionaries are not in the business of offering statistical data, they also do not attempt to define obesity in terms of numbers or formulae. That job has been taken up by insurance companies, medical experts, fitness professionals, and research scientists, who have all offered different numerical definitions of obesity based on different criteria at different times. The current standard definition used by most researchers is something called the Body Mass Index (BMI). Recommended by the World Health Organization and the National Institutes of Health (NIH), BMI is calculated by multiplying weight in pounds by 703, and dividing the result by the square of height in inches. For example, a five-foot-four-inch woman weighing 155 pounds (about the U.S. average) has a BMI of 26.6 as indicated by the following figures: 108,965 (155 times 703) divided by 4,096 (64 inches times 64) = 26.6 BMI. According to current U.S. government guidelines a BMI between 18.5 and 24.9 is considered normal; BMIs between 25.0 and 29.9 are considered overweight; a BMI of 30.0 or over is considered obese. A BMI under 18.5 is deemed underweight. Translated into pounds, a five-foot-four-inch woman would be considered to have a normal BMI if she weighed between 108 and 145 pounds. If she weighed between 145 and 174 pounds she would be considered overweight, and anything over 174 pounds would classify her as obese. The average BMI of U.S. adults is a little over 26, which means that the average U.S. adult is considered overweight. More than one-half of all men and women in America— roughly 118 million—are classified as either overweight or obese by current U.S. government-endorsed criteria.

Other definitions of obesity used at various times, now and in the past, are "20 percent or more over 'ideal' weight," "20 percent or more over 'normal' or average weight," "20 to 30 percent or more over the midpoint of the recommended weight range," and, as will be discussed below, a body fat percentage (of total body composition) of 20 to 25 percent for men, 30 to 35 percent for women. Sometimes obesity is a stage beyond merely "overweight" on the weight continuum. The current U.S. government guidelines are a perfect example. A five-foot-four-inch woman is "overweight" if she weighs 174 pounds (BMI = 29.9), but "obese" if she weighs 175 pounds (BMI = 30.1). A five-foot-ten-inch man is "overweight" at 208 pounds (BMI = 29.9), but "obese" at 209 pounds (BMI = 30.1)—despite the fact that body *fat* is not even measured.

The association between poor health and obesity has a venerable tradition, going back at least twenty-four centuries to the time of Hippocrates, the "Father of Western Medicine." Until quite recent times, though, overweight as a health risk was usually assumed to be relevant only to the very few at the far end of the "heavy" side of the bell-shaped weight-for-height distribution curve. Prior to this past century, excessive thinness was viewed as a potentially much greater threat to health than excessive fatness, since thin people appeared to be more vulnerable to two of the three diseases that were the most common killers of the time: tuberculosis and pneumonia. (Influenza was the third.) An ample supply of fat stores was looked upon as a sign of robust health. Not so anymore. The benign view of body fat changed dramatically in the twentieth century. No longer considered an indicator of vitality, of reserves that could be drawn upon, body fat began to be seen as an encumbrance that cut life short.

The negative perception of obesity that is so widespread in America today stems directly from events that took place in the life insurance industry in the early 1900s. In an effort to maximize their profits, the life insurance companies were looking for ways to screen applicants for their policies. If they could determine which variables were associated with premature mortality, they could charge higher premiums to those who had those risk factors, or refuse to insure them at all. Because weight was a variable that could be measured easily and inexpensively, the insurance companies' physicians, medical directors, and statisticians began assessing the data they had collected on their policyholders over the years to see if there was any relationship between mortality and body weight. Thus was born the insurance industry's height-weight table, which, from its earliest appearance in 1897 to its latest in 1983, was intended to serve as some kind of gauge of mortality risk.

When the first insurance industry-generated height-weight tables were published between the years 1897 and 1912, they were sex- and age-specific tables of the "average" weight of policyholders, who ranged in age from about fifteen to seventy. For a five-foot-four-inch woman, for example, average weight was 126 pounds at age twenty to twenty-nine,

132 at thirty to thirty-nine, 140 at forty to forty-nine, 145 at fifty to fifty-nine, and 144 at sixty to sixty-nine. Though "average" was what was recommended, and overweight was defined as *anything* over that weight range, the consensus was that mortality did not increase appreciably until one got to at least 20 percent over the average weight. Consequently, only those whose weights were 20 percent or more above average were required to pay higher premiums. In subsequent times, as will be discussed below, the weights at which risk supposedly set in would drop, and the national hysteria about weight as a health problem would rise accordingly. But this was the beginning of our national preoccupation with weight—and with weight tables. Our conviction that these tables tell us something significant about weight has not been diminished by the fact that the numbers on the insurance company tables have changed dramatically over the years, or that every five years since 1980 the U.S. government issued its own tables with its own figures, which varied with each edition and differed from those put out by the insurance industry.

Once the first tables had been created, the life insurance companies began spreading the gospel of the truth it thought was revealed by these tables with a moral fervor that went beyond the mere assessment of insurance risk. Believing that their findings could be the foundation not just of a more profitable industry but a of healthier nation, the medical directors of these companies began championing the weight-loss cause in speeches before medical societies and in articles written for both scientific and lay audiences. An early and eloquent example of this campaign to convert an industry concern to a national health agenda appeared in an article written by Dr. Brandreth Symonds, chief medical director of Mutual Life Insurance of New York, in the January 1909 issue of *McClure's*, a general-interest magazine. Based on an address he had earlier given to a group of physicians at the New Jersey Medical Society, Dr. Symonds's article stated that "excessive weight, whether it be fat or muscle, is not a storehouse of reserve strength, but a burden that has to be nourished, if muscle, and that markedly interferes with nutrition and function, if fat." Weight control, he advised physicians, was "the sermon which you should preach to your patients." Americans, he claimed, must be taught the health value of keeping body weight as close to the "average" (for their height, age, and gender) as possible. For its part, the Metropolitan Life Insurance Company established a Welfare Division and conducted numerous educational programs on public health. By 1943, its seventy-fifth year in business, it had distributed 1.2 billion pieces of health-related literature.

At the same time that the life insurance industry began issuing its dire warnings about the health implications of body fat, changes taking place within the fashion world only heightened the new fat phobia. In 1908 French designer Paul Poiret introduced a new, body-revealing style for women. His hobble-skirted dresses and slim sheaths placed a premium on slenderness—a dramatic departure from historical trends. Articles in *Vogue* and in other fashion magazines highlighted the new sleek look, which metamorphosed after World War I into the boyish, flapper look. Within a short time women's fashions had been completely transformed, and their bodies were apparently expected to follow suit. In effect two completely unrelated industries—life insurance and fashion—had by chance delivered two simultaneous and mutually reinforcing messages to the American public: Body fat is unfashionable as well as unhealthy.

Soon the new self-consciousness about body weight would be reflected in a proliferation of articles in the popular press. According to the *Reader's Guide to Periodical Literature*, between 1890 and 1909 only twelve articles were published on the subject of obesity (or "corpulence," as every edition of the *Reader's Guide* until 1977 referred to it). During the next two decades, however, more than one hundred articles appeared, bearing such titles as "New Methods of Flesh Reduction" (Harper's Bazaar, 1909), "Get Rid of That Fat" (*Saturday Evening Post*, 1917), and "Perils of Fatness" and "Fat and Fatality" (*Literary Digest*, 1921 and 1926 respectively). Though the consensus was not yet unanimous, most of the articles spread the word that weight control was a worthy goal, even if not a matter of life and death. Responding to the message, Americans now embarked on their first round of dieting mania. The powerful combination of health and vanity concerns had made them converts to the new ideal of thinness.

Initially, however, the medical profession itself was not nearly as enthusiastic. In the first place most doctors were still seeing a good many patients with diseases for which thinness seemed to be a primary risk factor. Secondly, according to the actuarial statistics cited by Dr. Symonds, one had to weigh at least 20 to 30 percent above average before experiencing an appreciable increase in mortality. At the time, the number of men and women who fell into this category was relatively small (at least among those who were policyholders). As a consequence, being overweight was not seen as a widespread public health problem. Just over three decades later, however, this perception would change dramatically— not because of a correspondingly dramatic change in Americans' body weight but because of a new definition of "too heavy."

This new statistical definition, courtesy of the Metropolitan Life Insurance Company, in effect *created* the obesity epidemic in the United States when new height-weight tables appeared in Met Life's journal, the *Statistical Bulletin*, a serious publication read mainly by insurance-company personnel, as well as people in the medical field. New tables for women were published in the October 1942 issue and those for men in June 1943. There were several important ways in which these tables and their figures differed from all the previous ones. First, the new weights given were not average but "ideal" weights. Second, the weights for a given height no longer varied by age; the "ideal" for all was the weight range associated with lowest mortality in twenty- to twenty-nine-year-olds. Third, though the weights for a given height did not vary by age, they did vary by frame size (small, medium, and large).

"Overweight: America's Number-One Health Problem"

These new weight standards were largely the inspiration of Louis I. Dublin, chief statistician for Met Life. The driving force within the company, Dublin had an unshakable belief in Met Life's actuarial data, which he himself helped to shape from the time he began working there in 1909 to the time of his death, at eighty-six, in 1969. Dublin spent much of his career trying to convince Americans that the greatest threat to their health was being overweight. To spread this message, he delivered countless speeches to a wide variety of audiences and wrote prolifically for both scientific journals and popular magazines. As far as changing public attitudes toward weight, he was probably the most influential person of the twentieth century. Of all his endeavors, none would have such long-lasting effect as the new "ideal weight" tables he persuaded Met Life to publish in the early 1940s.

Until then life insurance tables had suggested that the *best* weight to strive for was the average weight for one's height, age, and gender. Now, however, with the elimination of the age variable, Met Life was delivering the message that it was not okay to gain weight with age. Looking at the data on hundreds of thousands of policyholders, Dublin and his fellow Met Life statistician, Herbert Marks, had observed that relatively modest increases over average weight in those over the age of thirty were associated with increases in mortality; therefore, they assumed, the average weights of people in their twenties were the ideal weights people should strive to maintain throughout life.

The result for that five-foot-four-inch "average" woman we've been talking about is that she was probably overweight once she left her twenties—unless she was in the large-frame group. A small-frame five-foot-four-inch woman was supposed to weigh 116-125; a medium-frame, 124-132; and a large frame, 131-142. Thus, if she was in the 30-39 age group and had attained the average weight of 132, she was at the outer edge of acceptable. If she was in the 40-49 age group and attained the average weight of 140, she was close to being overweight even in the large-frame range. By redefining what was average as "too fat," the new tables diagnosed a supposed weight problem in at least one-half of adult Americans, despite the fact that Americans' average weight had not changed appreciably since the turn of the century.

To fortify the message that weight control "is more urgent than ever before," Met Life pulled out all the stops. Claiming that adult weight gain over the years was principally the result of overeating, the *Statistical Bulletin* called upon Americans to eat less. This was an appeal not just to their health concerns but also to their patriotism. Consuming less would free up more food "to properly feed our fighting men.... Overeating, which even in peacetime is an indefensible habit of self-indulgence, is little short of scandalous today." As if gluttony weren't bad enough, the "self-indulgence" of those whom Met Life had defined as overweight now apparently bordered on treason.

Issues of patriotism aside, Met Life's single-minded focus on "overeating" as the cause for weight gain in adult men and women had the unfortunate effect of deflecting attention from another possible cause:

under-exercising. Though the *Statistical Bulletin* did acknowledge that weight gain reflected "the effect of persisting in the habit of consuming the same amount of food while physical activity decreases," there was no corresponding emphasis on changing the sedentary lifestyle. (That issue would not be addressed until 1959, when Met Life issued the next generation of weight tables and finally began to advocate exercise as an advisable component of a weight-loss program.)

In the years to come, Met Life would gradually win the medical establishment over to its views. Since medicine was coming into its Golden Age at this time, with respect for physicians at an all-time high, the timing of this latest salvo in its weight-loss campaign could not have been better. Doctors in key positions around the country began to "preach" the "sermon" Dr. Symonds had urged upon them at the beginning of the century. Obesity, and the overeating that was assumed to be its cause, were "a waste of our national resources not only in manpower but in food," Dr. James M. Hundley of the National Institute of Arthritis and Metabolic Diseases announced to a group of physicians and nutritionists in Chicago in 1951. A year later Dr. W. H. Sebrell, Jr., then director of the National Institutes of Health, proclaimed obesity "the number one nutritional problem in the United States." These refrains, and variations on them, would be repeated ceaselessly for years to come. The efforts of Louis Dublin and his fellow life insurance medical directors were finally paying off.

The turning point came in 1951. That was the year the campaign against obesity was taken up by the U.S. government and the medical establishment. Joining forces with the life insurance industry, the American Medical Association (AMA) and the United States Public Health Service embarked upon "a nationwide effort...to stimulate interest anew in the problem of obesity and to spur positive action against it." At the annual meeting of the AMA in Atlantic City in June of that year, the joint effort was unveiled in the course of a special symposium on overweight, nutrition, and health. Overweight was targeted as the "outstanding" factor responsible for the degenerative diseases—for example, cardiovascular and kidney diseases, cancer, and diabetes—that were now identified as the leading causes of death. "Taking off excess weight" was identified as a critical remedy for these ills.

To facilitate the immediate and widespread dissemination of this message, Met Life's Health and Welfare Division had created a number audiences and including everything from slide shows and pamphlets to the nationwide theatrical release of a short movie on losing weight entitled *Cheers for Chubby*. The exclusive emphasis on caloric restriction continued to characterize the weight-loss campaign. Exercise as well as drug remedies should be recommended only with discretion, physicians were advised, because they were "entirely secondary to diet" as a remedy "and may divert patient's attention from his main problem, which is overeating." Since many of the myriad pharmacological remedies for obesity that had been introduced in that century had serious, sometimes even fatal consequences, it was certainly the better part of wisdom to preach caution against the use of drugs (even though that wasn't the reason cited for minimizing their use). But it was too bad that exercise was considered just as "secondary" to the agenda as drugs were.

Given that diet was the key weapon in the battle, it was natural that nutritionists were called upon to join the campaign. Quick to enlist, they soon became a major force in the weight-loss industry. Weight control, not nutrition *per se*, is what most nutritionists today perceive as their primary mission. This was made perfectly clear in a survey published in the September 1991 issue of *Prevention* magazine. More than three hundred of the top nutrition experts in the United States were asked to rate forty-four different nutritional changes they might recommend to their clients. Ninety-seven percent of the experts indicated that controlling weight by controlling calorie intake was their highest priority. A decade later nothing has changed. The annual meetings of the American Dietetics Association are dominated by a "weight-loss" mentality. Little more than lip service is paid to alternative, nondiet approaches to health.

Just as had happened earlier in the century, the weight-loss campaign was given additional ballast by the fashion industry, a process that began in 1947 and has never really let up since. In that year, Christian Dior introduced his "New Look" for women's clothing, and in so doing stunned the fashion world. Champion of the seventeen-inch waist for women, which was impossible for all but a very few, generally very young women, Dior had created the "épée silhouette"—slender as a fencing blade, as *Newsweek* described it to American audiences. Though there was at first considerable resistance to the look, with many women rebelling against the corsets Dior expected them to wear to achieve his wasp-waisted ideal, the New Look gradually prevailed. Department store mannequins tell the story in a nutshell: until about 1950 their physical dimensions were similar to those of the women who bought the clothes they modeled. Since then, the dimensions have been shrinking, so that they now no longer bear any resemblance to the measurements of the average women. From Twiggy in the 1960s to Kate Moss in the 1990s, the same could be said for real-life models.

Ignoring the fact that the look being celebrated in the fashion press was completely unrealistic as a goal, no less an authority than Louis Dublin himself offered his praise in the July 1952 issue of *Reader's Digest*: "The effort to maintain a fashionable silhouette keeps women watching their weight and diet. The result has aided their health as well as their appearance." Furthermore, he lamented the fact that the forces of fashion had not inspired a similar effort in men.

Fuelled by the combined forces of the medical community, the federal government, the life insurance industry, and the world of fashion, the campaign for weight loss escalated at an exponential rate of growth; and the media delivered the message. In the 1950s the number of articles on weight averaged about thirty per year—more than the total number published during the entire first half of the century. Nearly four hundred more articles devoted specifically to "diet" were published during this same pivotal period of the campaign. In contrast to the articles on diet that had been published in previous times, these were not about healthy, nutritious eating, but rather about losing weight. Books joined the same trend. Midway through the twentieth century only a modest number of books on obesity and dieting had found their way into print. In early 2002 Amazon.com listed more than 16,000 titles under the key word "diet," and more than 600 for "obesity."

Recommended Weights Drop Again

In 1959, the weight control cause received yet another boost with the publication of the massive Build and Blood Pressure Study conducted by the Society of Actuaries and Association of Life Insurance Medical Directors of America. What made this study unique was its scale:

Twenty-six life insurance companies in Canada and the United States had pooled the data on 4.9 million policyholders to further the research on weight and longevity. The conclusion it reached was basically the same as that of earlier studies: Higher weights were associated with poor health and shortened life spans. Shortly after its release the study was lauded as the most definitive and persuasive proof to date that obesity was killing Americans. Armed with this massive set of data, Met Life now issued another table of recommended weights—now called "desirable" rather than "ideal"—which were even lower than before. The new weight standards indicated that our five-foot-four-inch woman with a small frame should weigh 108-116 (down from 116-125 in 1942); with a medium frame she should weigh 113-126 (down from 124-132); and with a large frame 121-138 (down from 131-142). The obesity epidemic had experienced yet another dramatic surge, which was once again caused mainly by a decrease in what Americans were being told to weigh, rather than an increase in what they actually weighed.

Fashion had done such a good job on women that they weighed a bit less on average by two to four pounds. Men, however, did weigh a bit more—one to four pounds. Perhaps this was why the redesigned weight control campaign Met Life embarked on at this juncture had a new component. Although limiting calorie intake remained the cornerstone, there was one important addition: exercise. Met Life was now recommending physically active recreation and regular exercise to the American public. Since decades of urging reduced calorie intake had apparently not been sufficient to reduce male waistlines, maybe exercise would do the job. Again the timing of Met Life's new campaign was perfect. It fit right in with trends that had gotten under way in the mid-1950s.

This was an era when Americans had become greatly alarmed by studies showing that European children far outperformed American children on fitness tests. In June 1956 President Eisenhower announced the formation of the President's Council on Youth Fitness (now called the President's Council on Physical Fitness and Sports) and a President's Citizens Advisory Committee on the Fitness of American Youth. These organizations set in motion a fitness movement that has held the imagination of the American public to the present day. (How much it has actually changed American habits is quite another issue.) The active, vigorous, touch-football-playing Kennedy's, who occupied center stage of American life after John F. Kennedy was inaugurated in 1961, gave the movement yet another boost.

By the end of the 1960s *aerobics* had been added to the American lexicon. Its *Webster's Dictionary* definition called it "a system of physical conditioning involving exercises strenuously performed." But it had become more than an exercise system; it was a new ethos promising a fat-free body. Exercise was not just a means to physical fitness but another weapon in the arsenal with which we were attacking obesity. Within a very short time "fitness" would come to be viewed as the polar opposite of "fatness."

The Antifat Movement

No better example of this new approach can be found than Covert Bailey's classic book, *Fit or Fat?*, which has been a favorite among fitness buffs and a perennial bestseller ever since its publication in the 1970s. One has only to look at the title to understand the core message of the book: A person can be fit *or* fat, but not both. It also implies that fat is the enemy, not overweight *per se*, which may be acceptable if a higher than usual proportion of that "excess" poundage is made up of muscle and bone. For nearly three decades, *Fit or Fat?* has been reinforcing the negative perception of body fat, attacking it, rather than weight, as the problem. Bailey and the thousands of other fitness experts who share his views distinguish "overfat," which is defined in terms of a given percentage of overall body composition, from "overweight," which simply means being heavier than the standards suggested by the height-weight tables. Just as some medical and life insurance company experts may distinguish between overweight and obesity, the difference being one of degree, so, too, do some of the people in the fitness establishment make a similar distinction between overfat and obesity, based on degree. The two respective sets of terms are also often used interchangeably, so that it can be difficult to pin down what any given use of one of those words may mean.

However, the concept of "overfat," whatever it means from context to context, is now firmly entrenched, and body fat percentage is regarded by many experts as one of the best criteria of fitness. Indeed, so much emphasis has been placed on this measurement that an assessment of body fat percentage—via caliper, underwater immersion test, or more high-tech means such as ultrasound and bioelectrical impedance (a measure of electrical resistance in the body)—has become a routine part of fitness evaluations. In many instances the measure of body fat has become the *sole* criterion for fitness. In the same way that it is possible to be overweight but not overfat, the exercise professionals say, it is possible to be within or even below the acceptable range as dictated by height-weight tables and yet be "overfat" because of an excess of fat (adipose) tissue. They assume that body fat is bad and that lean tissue, such as muscle, is good. The fact is some fat can be healthy fat, just as some muscle can be unhealthy. The quality of the tissue has to be considered.

The body fat determinations share the same problem that the height-weight tables have. Although body fat percentages can be measured almost as easily and accurately as height and weight, what do they mean? The concept of "overfat" is of little value unless its impact on health and longevity can be quantified. While high percentages of body fat may be *associated* with poor health or decreased longevity, rigorous statistical examination of data actually reveals a relatively weak correlation, suggesting that very little, if any, of the poor health or decreased longevity observed in obese people can actually be explained by body fat (an issue that will be explored in-depth in Chapter 3). This problem has not deterred the fitness professionals. Despite the fact that there are no valid guidelines for determining what percentage of fat is compatible with being fit or healthy, recommended body fat standards have been set, the consensus being that something like 15 percent of total body composition should be made up of fat in men, 22 percent in women. (I say "something like" because these percentages do vary from expert to expert, and, as with weight tables, may reflect either "ideals" or "averages.") Because many exercise scientists specializing in body composition work with athletes, the body fat standards for the population as a whole tended to be developed with the athlete in mind, on the assumption that athletes are healthy in part because of their generally low body fat percentages.

Relatively few Americans meet the 15 and 22 percent standards, however, especially once they are out of their twenties; between 75 and 90 percent of middle-aged men and women in the United States exceed the recommendations. But just as Dr. Dublin and Met Life decreed that no increase in weight was supposed to occur with age, the fitness establishment has decreed that increases in body fat are similarly undesirable and unjustifiable.

Obesity is defined as anything over about 20 to 25 percent body fat for men, 30 to 35 percent body fat for women. By these criteria, and depending on age, somewhere between 20 and 65 percent of men and women in America are obese or "overfat." With the use of these arbitrary measurements, which have never been tied to objective assessments of body fat as a *causal* factor in either higher disease or higher mortality rates, the exercise scientists have created an obesity epidemic of their own, comparable to, if not statistically identical with, that created by the insurance industry.

Staying the Course

By the early 1980s the weight control campaign had acquired so much momentum that nothing could stop it. Indeed it would prove difficult even to change its course slightly, as Met Life discovered when it set off a massive public debate with its publication of new tables that reversed the previous trend toward ever lower recommended weights. Although Met Life's *Statistical Bulletin* stressed that "it is better to be lean than to be plump, and wiser to weigh less than the average rather than more," the new weight standards were *heavier* than those in 1959 were. The five-foot-four-inch woman who, in 1959, was advised to weigh between 108 and 116 if she was small of frame could now weigh 114-127; the medium-frame woman whose weight in 1959 was set at 113-126 was now upped to 124-138; and the large-frame woman was allowed an increase from 121-138 to 134-151. Short men and women seem to have benefited most, with the average increases in allowable weight on the order of 10 to 13 pounds. Men and women of average or taller weight were allowed an extra 2 to 8 pounds. Because the most recent actuarial data, from the 1979 Build Study, indicated that the best weights for longevity had increased by amounts up to 17 percent over what had been recommended a generation before, Met Life was now trying to reverse a tide that had been flowing in one direction—downward—since the beginning of the century.

Another aspect of the reversal had to do with the gap between the average weight of policyholders and the weight associated with lowest mortality. With the new data that gap appeared to have narrowed considerably, especially for women, where the difference between recommended and average was just a few pounds. The earlier insistence that "ideal" or "desirable" weight was well below average weight no longer seemed justified. Being about average, it now appeared, was not so bad after all.

Perhaps because the new weight standards were such a challenge to the trend Met Life itself had helped create, the message accompanying their release seemed almost to be trying to minimize their significance:

> They are not the weights that minimize illness or the incidence of disease. Neither are they the weights that optimize job per-formance, nor the weights for best appearance. Because the words "ideal" and "desirable" mean different things to different people and have created confusion, these terms will no longer be used in referring to Metropolitan's height and weight tables. No one standard of weights can always satisfy the needs of the public, the medical profession, public health workers, or nutritionists, nor can such a standard necessarily be appropriate for those suf-fering from various impairments or disease.

The sweeping indictment of overweight that had characterized decades of antiobesity propaganda had been softened. All that Met Life was now willing to claim for its new tables was that they, "like the earlier tables, simply indicate the weights at which people should have the greatest longevity," for they were "based on the lowest mortality for men and women at ages 25 to 59...." One has to wonder, though, just how much confidence Met Life had in this claim. Despite maintaining that the tables reflect weights associated with lowest mortality, the company apparently doesn't even use them. That's right. Amidst all the other conclusions downplaying the significance of the tables it had created, Met Life dropped this bombshell: "These weights are not used for underwriting or in the computation of premiums."

While the tone was softened, the core of the message remained the same, which should have made the change easier to accept. Unfortunately, Met Life couldn't seem to induce a similar modulation of tone in the rest of the health establishment. The revised weight standards came under attack by many leaders in the fields of health care and nutrition, who simply did not believe the new actuarial data. The medical and scientific communities continued to publish hundreds of papers in their journals in which the battle against weight was maintained at the same high pitch, and the words *ideal* and *desirable* continued to be applied to various weight recommendations.

In 1985 a U.S. government-sponsored conference on the "Health Implications of Obesity," under the aegis of the National Institutes of Health, may even have taken the battle to a new level of intensity. Though the panel's scientists issued a rather clinical and familiar-sounding statement about how "obesity, defined as excessive storage of energy in the form of fat, has adverse effects on health and longevity," the story got sensationalized by such newspaper headlines as "Obesity is 'Killer Disease' Affecting 34 Million Americans, NIH Reports" and "Panel Finds Obesity a Major U.S. Killer." The fact that experts at the conference presented a large amount of data that questioned the prevailing assumptions about weight, health, and longevity did not find its way into the popular press, nor was that material reflected in the panel's "consensus" statement (as will be discussed in the next chapter).

Thus was a new beachhead established in the war on obesity. The idea that obesity is not just a cause of disease but a disease itself has gained widespread acceptance, and the NIH panel's concluding statement has been consistently cited as justification for continuing the war on body fat.

At the present time, however, body fat seems to be winning, as Americans continue to get fatter, not thinner. Between 1980 and 1991, for example, the ranks of the overweight and obese (i.e., BMI of 25 or greater) swelled by nearly 31 percent, from about 78 million adults aged eighteen to seventy-four to 102 million. Currently more than one-half of U.S. adults—56.4 percent, or approximately 118 million based on 2000 census data—are now considered either overweight or obese, according to an article that appeared in the September 12, 2001, issue of the *Journal of the American Medical Association*. About 40 million of this total—nearly one out of every five U.S. adults—are classified as obese (BMI of 30 or greater). The increase in the average weight of U.S. adults during the past two decades is about 15 pounds—this despite the fact that virtually every major medical and health organization still trumpets the battle cry against fat. While some modulating voices are beginning to be heard, we are still inclined to listen to the more strident messages. Those at the vanguard of the weight-loss crusade are now saying that Americans should strive for a weight at least 10 to 15 percent below average (reminiscent of the Met Life standards of the 1940s and 1950s). By those standards at least 75 percent of adult Americans are too fat.

Again we must ask, *Too fat for what?* Good health? A long life? Although the antiobesity warriors are convinced, and have done a good job of convincing us, that weight loss itself improves health and lengthens life, there are absolutely no studies that unequivocally show this to be true. In fact, many studies indicate that voluntary weight loss may compromise health and increase risk for premature death. All these studies, on both sides of the issue, have to be carefully examined so that we can distinguish between connections that appear to be causal, but may be merely associative.

Can a century's worth of assumptions about obesity be wrong? Do millions of Americans risk premature death *unless* they lose weight—or *because* they lose weight? Part Two will help to assess the validity of the long-fought battle against obesity.

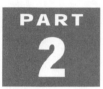

PART 2

EXPOSING THE MYTHS

CHAPTER 3

Is Obesity a Killer Disease?
A Closer Look at the Evidence

The available data do not support the hypothesis that obesity causes atherosclerosis.
—Elizabeth Barrett-Conner, M.D., University of California at San Diego School of Medicine, from "Obesity, Atherosclerosis, and Coronary Artery Disease," a paper she gave at the Health Implications of Obesity Conference, in Bethesda, MD, 1985

If obesity is a killer disease, as the chairman of the Obesity Conference told newspaper reporters in 1985, and one that affects tens of millions of Americans, then we might reasonably expect it to be implicated in atherosclerosis, or clogged arteries, which is the number-one killer in America. Not only do most data fail to support that hypothesis, but few of the available data support *any* of the numerous hypotheses about overweight as a primary cause of *any* of the major diseases for which it is routinely blamed (with the exception of osteoarthritis; more on this, and on the impact of weight on bone health in general, in Chapter 7). These hypotheses are, however, constantly being presented to us as facts.

The 1985 conference is a perfect example of how this process of distortion occurs. The NIH-sponsored meeting was one of a series of what are known as *consensus conferences*, at which state-of-the-art overviews of various health problems are presented by a series of experts in the field. A presumably impartial panel of scientists listens to the evidence from all sides and then drafts a "consensus statement" evaluating the evidence they have just heard.

At the conference Dr. Barrett-Conner cited dozens of scientific studies in support of her conclusion exonerating obesity as a cause of athero-sclerosis. Nor was she alone in her dissension from the conventional views. Dr. Reubin Andres, clinical director of the National Institute on Aging and a professor of medicine at Johns Hopkins, delivered a report based on an independent statistical analysis he had performed on the data from the 1979 Build Study. He found that, contrary to the popular wisdom (and the 1983 Met Life tables, which allowed for no weight gain over the years), the body weights associated with lowest mortality increased progressively with age. By the time a woman reaches her sixties, for example, the BMI associated with lowest mortality is 27.3—*overweight*, according to current BMI criteria.

About half of the seventeen other expert presenters also made statements that were not at all consistent with, and in some instances diametrically opposed to, the view that obesity *per se* "has adverse effects on health and longevity." That is a quote from the so-called "consensus" statement that was published after all the experts presented their data to the panel of scientists. In the *International Journal of Obesity*, where a scientific summation of the conference proceedings appeared, not a single one of the studies showing obesity to be harm-less got a mention, despite their having been cited at length and in detail by Dr. Barrett-Conner and a number of the other dissenting experts. Instead two-thirds of the cited references were from the life insurance companies' actuarial data—data that are seriously flawed (as will be explained in the next chapter). There was no acknowledgment whatsoever of Dr. Andres's dissenting assessment of that data.

Using a double standard for evaluating evidence, the fourteen scientists on the panel simply ignored all the data that contradicted what they believed. This is an example of what I call rounding up the usual suspects—obesity being the prime one. Nearly a century's worth of propaganda, reinforced by the fact that so many serious illnesses are so frequently found in people who are obese, made it impossible for the panel to render an impartial judgment. The guilt-by-association case against obesity had once again prevailed.

Perhaps this case is never made more convincingly than when obesity is on trial for causing heart disease—our deadliest killer, responsible for more deaths in the United States than any other disease. Obesity is supposedly guilty of causing clogged arteries and contributing to several of the major risk factors for cardiovascular disease: high blood pressure, high levels of blood fats (for example, LDL cholesterol, which is the "bad" cholesterol, and triglycerides), and type 2 diabetes. In reality, evidence presented in this chapter will show:

- Obesity is a very poor predictor of hypertension (high blood pressure).

- Obesity is a very poor predictor of high cholesterol and hyperlipidemia (high blood fats).

- Direct measures of atherosclerosis (clogged arteries) in a number of studies using a variety of techniques show obesity to be completely unrelated to the presence of this form of cardiovascular disease, or to the progression of this disease over time.

- Most people with type 2—non-insulin dependent—diabetes can so substantially improve their condition through changes in diet and exercise that, *even when they have lost little or no weight and remain at weights that are clinically obese*, they can discontinue their medications.

The obesity/heart disease hypothesis cannot stand up to the evidence.

Obesity and Its Relationship to High Blood Pressure

I've worked with hundreds of men and women over the past 10 years, who seem to me like living proof that obesity is a relatively neutral factor in matters of health. Most of the individuals I've encountered with high blood pressure have not been obese, and a good many obese people have not had high blood pressure. Countless research studies have confirmed what I've observed firsthand. Typically, over 85 percent of the variation in blood pressure within a population is found to have nothing to do with body fat. When you look at a graphic display of the data concerning the possible relationships, the results are nothing like a neat straight line on which ever-heavier weights correspond to ever-higher blood pressures. Instead, the results resemble a well-used dartboard, with random markings all over the place and a nearly complete lack of predictability. In reality, the accuracy of predicting a woman's blood pressure just by knowing her BMI is only about 15 percent better than just guessing.

Even though it is true that high blood pressure is more common in large persons compared to thin persons, body fat *per se* is probably not the culprit. Data from the second National Health and Nutrition Examination Survey (NHANES II), a U.S. government-sponsored study of over twenty thousand people during the years 1976 to 1980, indicated that *excess lean body tissue* is more strongly linked to high blood pressure than is excess body fat. In this study body fatness was defined in terms of commonly used skin fold thickness, and overweight was defined in terms of BMI alone. The study researchers created five classifications based on varying degrees of fatness and BMI:

- *Underweight and lean:* below the 15th percentile for both BMI and skin fold thickness;
- *Average weight and average fatness:* between the 15th and 85th percentiles for both BMI and skin fold thickness;
- *Obese but not overweight:* above the 85th percentile for skin fold thickness, but less than the 85th percentile for BMI;
- *Overweight but not obese:* above the 85th percentile for BMI, but less than the 85th percentile for skin fold thickness;
- *Overweight and obese:* above the 85th percentile for both skin fold thickness and BMI.

Men and women who were classified as "obese but not overweight" were only about one-third to one-half as likely to have high blood pressure as men and women classified as "overweight but not obese." Men and women classified as "obese but not overweight" were no more likely to have high blood pressure than men and women classified as either "average weight and average fatness" or "underweight and lean." These results strongly suggest that it is the excess "fat free" tissue of large people that may contribute to their blood pressure problems.

In support of these findings are the observations from several studies showing that the reduction in blood pressure associated with weight loss is more closely correlated to decreases in lean body mass than with changes in body fat.

Another potential explanation for the higher prevalence of hypertension among persons with high BMI is yo-yo dieting. A substantial body of evidence from animal studies shows that hypertension is linked more strongly to weight cycling (one of the preferred terms researchers use to characterize yo-yoing) than to obesity. Although this will be discussed in more detail in Chapter 7, one particularly relevant example on humans is worth mentioning now. Recently a group of Italian researchers compared blood pressures of 96 obese women who had a history of yo-yo dieting with 96 obese women who had no history of dieting. The women were between the ages of 25 and 45, and the two groups were the same in every respect measured—except two: dieting history and blood pressure. Weight cycling was defined as five or more weight losses of at least 10 pounds within the previous five years.

Blood pressure in the 96 women with no history of dieting averaged 125 over 79 millimeters of mercury pressure (125/79 mmHg)—very normal indeed, especially considering the fact that these women, at 195 pounds, were 60 pounds overweight by BMI standards. In comparison, the women with a history of yo-yoing had blood pressures that averaged 147/90 mmHg—which meets or exceeds the current clinical definition of hypertension (blood pressure equal to or greater than 140/90 mmHg). Since the two groups of women were similar in virtually all respects, including BMI (about 36), it is very likely that yo-yo dieting contributed to the difference in blood pressure. In fact, blood pressure was positively correlated with the total number of pounds that the yo-yoers reported they had regained after their multiple weight-loss attempts during the previous five years. Because weight loss via dieting is rarely maintained, and because dieting is more common among people of size, the association between obesity and hypertension may just reflect the fact that obese people yo-yo more.

Nonetheless, the standard advice to people with high blood pressure is: Lose weight. Or, to put it in the language of one study, "weight reduction [should be recommended] as a critical intervention in modifying risk." This statement is from the report issued by the Veterans

Administration Normative Aging Study, a fifteen-year examination of the possible effects of weight gain on risk factors for heart disease. Nearly fourteen hundred men in Boston, Massachusetts, were studied, and measurements of blood pressure as well as blood fats, uric acid, glucose, and other possible risk factors were taken to see if there was a correlation between changes in those variables and changes in recorded weights. Though only a small percentage—1 to 5 percent—of the change in any given risk factor for heart disease could be attributed to changes in body weight, the researchers still came to the conclusion that weight loss would be a "critical intervention."

This standard advice is not without consequences. The first problem, of course, is that few people who lose weight can keep it off, which means that doctors' advice often leads people into endless cycles of weight loss and gain, with results that can be extremely detrimental to health, and in some cases even fatal (as will be discussed in Chapter 7). The second possible repercussion is more fundamental to the obesity/disease hypothesis: Among those with high blood pressure, weight loss, even if maintained, may not resolve the problem.

Perhaps the fact that weight loss may not always alleviate hypertension doesn't seem like a good argument against weight loss. After all, if it alleviates it in *some* cases, then that should be reason enough to recommend it. However, a well-documented but rarely acknowledged observation about hypertension is that *in obese people it only marginally increases the risk of premature death*. The reverse applies to both nonobese and thin people, for whom hypertension more than doubles the risk of premature mortality. Evidence for this has existed for more than forty years and has been confirmed by recent studies in the United States and France. So, if a hypertensive obese person follows the advice to lose weight in order to lower blood pressure and the remedy doesn't work, then what you have is a weight-reduced hypertensive who is now statistically more likely to die from cardiovascular disease than before. This may help explain the seemingly inexplicable finding in so many studies that men and women who have undergone sustained weight loss are at greater risk of cardiovascular disease mortality than others. Sometimes it appears that it's not just cardiovascular disease mortality rates that increase with weight loss accompanied by elevations in blood pressure, but mortality from all causes. Ironic as it may seem, it might be more prudent to tell thin hypertensives to gain a few pounds than to advise heavy ones to lose.

Take the famous Framingham Heart Study, which will be described in detail in the next chapter. A 1993 article in the *Annals of Internal Medicine* reported on a study of the results of weight change in twenty-five hundred of the men and women from Framingham, Massachusetts, representing about half the original population database of the study. Their weight was assessed six years after the 1948 starting date for the study, when the subjects were between the ages of thirty-five and fifty-four, and it was assessed every two years over the next ten years, as was blood pressure. Some people lost weight over the ten years, some gained, and some stayed weight stable. Surprisingly, *both* the weight gainers and the weight losers showed increases in blood pressure and in the incidence of hypertension; more predictably, the blood pressure increases in the weight gainers were greater, almost by twofold. However, that didn't seem to have any bearing on death rates.

During a twenty-year follow-up to the initial ten-year period, when the relationship between weight gain, increased blood pressure, and mortality rates was assessed, the results were quite complicated and in many ways unexpected. In men, for example, despite the much greater increase in blood pressure among the weight gainers, there was no comparable increase in mortality rates. Among men, the weight gainers had mortality rates from heart disease that were 50 percent lower than the weight losers (and somewhat lower even than those who were weight stable)—suggestive of the notion that increases in blood pressure and in the incidence of hypertension were *not* detrimental in weight gainers, but were in weight losers. Moreover, the weight gainers had all-cause mortality rates that were 41 percent lower than the weight losers.

For women, the results were murkier. Suffice it to say that weight gain didn't seem to adversely affect their mortality rates, even though the weight gainers experienced increases in blood pressure that were twice those of the weight losers, and a higher incidence of hypertension also. Conversely, weight losers had a 38 percent higher mortality rate than those who were weight stable.

Why hypertension is a relatively benign factor in obese people is a question still being investigated, but the answer seems to have something to do with the fact that the obese hypertensive's vascular system is not stressed in the same manner as that of the nonobese hypertensive. To understand how this might be the case we have to understand what hypertension is. As indicated by its popular name, high blood pressure, it is a condition in which the blood exerts a greater than normal pressure against the walls of the blood vessels.

There are two factors involved in blood pressure: cardiac output and peripheral vascular resistance. Cardiac output is the total amount of blood that is pumped from the heart, and peripheral resistance is the amount of resistance to the blood flow within the body's entire system of arteries. Elevations in either or both of these factors can cause blood pressure to rise, but generally speaking it is raised peripheral vascular resistance that is seen as the guilty party in cardiovascular disease. Since heavy people generally have higher cardiac output than thin people, an obese hypertensive with the same blood pressure as a thin hypertensive is likely to have a lower vascular resistance, which means a less stressed vascular system and lower risk of cardiovascular disease. The equation for blood pressure measurement, Resistance multiplied by Cardiac Output, $BP = R \times CO$, explains why this is true, for a higher cardiac output multiplied by a lower resistance (as in a fat person) can end up creating the same blood pressure as a lower cardiac output multiplied by a higher resistance (as in a thin person).

Another possible explanation for the elevated cardiovascular disease risk of lean hypertensives is that lean people with high blood pressure secrete about two and one-half times the amount of stress hormones, such as adrenaline, in response to exercise as compared with obese people with equally high blood pressure. Researchers at the State University of New York, Downstate Medical Center in Brooklyn, who reported the findings in the January 2001 issue of the *Journal of the American College of Cardiology*, concluded that the exaggerated stress hormone response in lean hypertensives may explain their "poorer cardiovascular prognosis."

While high blood pressure in obese people cannot be dismissed as a matter for concern, especially since it may be a sign of other physical problems, its seriousness seems more often to be lessened, rather than increased, by overweight.

Obesity and Its Relationship to Atherosclerosis

Atherosclerosis occurs when there is a buildup of fatty plaque on the walls of the arteries, which eventually narrows the passage through which the blood flows. It is both an effect and a cause of hypertension because, when fat-clogged blood vessels are subjected to high blood pressure over a long period of time, they become rigid and inflexible—a process called "hardening of the arteries." The narrowing and stiffening then contribute to additional increases in blood pressure. Atherosclerosis of the arteries in the heart can damage the heart and might lead to fatal heart attacks. Depending on where the buildups of fatty deposits are located, atherosclerosis can also cause strokes, blood clots, and many other serious problems.

Because obese people have more fat on their bodies, it has been assumed that they must also have more fat in their arteries. If this were true, then we should be able to predictably connect weight in general, or body fat in particular, to atherosclerosis and the progression of this disease over time, but the fact is we can't. There are three categories of research to prove this: autopsy studies, coronary angiography studies, and ultrasound studies.

What Autopsies Tell Us about Obesity and Atherosclerosis

Studies done on the bodies of people who had coronary disease provide a very direct means of assessing whether weight or body fat correlates to atherosclerosis. Studies of this nature date back at least to the 1940s, and the methodology they employed was aptly described by Dr. Ancel Keys, of the University of Minnesota, in 1954. As explained by Dr. Keys (who was also responsible for what I believe to have been the first controlled "yo-yo dieting" experiment): "We take each person for whom a reliable diagnosis of coronary disease is made and measure him to see if he is fat or thin, or express his body weight as a percentage of the average for healthy persons of the same height and age." Many such studies were conducted in the 1940s and early 1950s, with results that were consistent and surprising: Neither weight nor body fat was related to atherosclerosis.

Evidence from similar autopsy studies done in this country, as well as in others, has been pouring in ever since the 1950s. Men and women, black and white, have all been autopsied, and always with the same result—the finding that "obesity itself is not an atherogenic agent." This statement came from Dr. Yogesh Patel of the Louisiana State University Medical Center, who headed up a research team that did autopsy analyses of 1,320 black and Caucasian men in New Orleans.

Even massively obese men and women show no connection between obesity and vascular disease. NIH researchers Drs. Carole Warnes and William Roberts published a report in 1984 describing the autopsy findings on men and women who weighed between three hundred and five hundred pounds at the time of death. There was no more atherosclerosis in their coronary vessels than in nonobese people of the same age.

Perhaps the most definitive of the autopsy studies was the International Atherosclerosis Project, which began collecting autopsy results in 1960 and eventually evaluated the coronary arteries from twenty-three thousand people in fourteen different countries. The number of specimens analyzed, and the broad spectrum of ethnic groups and geographic locations from which they were drawn, made this study unique in its comprehensiveness. When the results of this landmark study were summarized by twenty-three physicians and scientists in an article published in 1968, the finding was unequivocal: "No association was found between several measures of obesity, body weight, body height, and trunk length with atherosclerosis."

For more than five decades, autopsy studies have been consistently delivering results that say that obesity does not cause heart disease, but the evidence they have produced has been ignored. Why? Is it once again a matter of ignoring those results that don't fall into line with the prevailing ideology? Or is it that these studies haven't gotten the attention they should because many of them are viewed as being dated, their technology old-fashioned? If the latter, then the state-of-the-art equipment used in today's coronary angiography studies should dispel any doubts about the autopsy findings, because this most sophisticated of scientific methods is coming up with similar results.

What Angiography Tells Us about Obesity and Atherosclerosis

Coronary angiography is without question the most sensitive and specific method available for assessing coronary artery disease, and it is used on living persons, not cadavers. This powerful technology involves a catheter being inserted into the aorta, and then into the heart itself, through which a dye is infused into the bloodstream that flows through the coronary arteries. An X-ray picture of the heart and associated blood vessels is then taken so that the cardiologist can assess the location and extent of any atherosclerosis.

Angiographic studies fall into two basic types. In the first type a cross-section of a particular population is evaluated on a one-time-only basis. A variety of body fat and body weight measurements assess the degree of obesity; the angiogram measures the extent of coronary atherosclerosis; and a statistical analysis is then done to see if there is any correlation between obesity and heart disease. Other risk factors, behavioral as well as biochemical, are also evaluated and analyzed for possible connections to atherosclerosis. In the second type of study, angiograms are performed not once but twice or more, over a period of several months or years, and the other measurements and analyses are also done at the same time; if there is any progression of the disease, it can be monitored and possible connections to that progression can be assessed.

Both types of studies yield the same results. Angiographic analysis invariably shows that the other risk factors—smoking, hypertension, elevated blood-fat levels, and diabetes—*are* related to atherosclerosis. In contrast, well over half of the angiographic studies that were done between 1976 and 2000 showed obesity to have *no* relationship to either the presence of atherosclerosis or the progression of this disease over time. One of the one-time-only studies showed something even more surprising.

A research team headed up by Dr. William Applegate of the University of Tennessee examined angiograms from over forty-five hundred middle-aged and elderly men and women—the largest, most comprehensive investigation of its kind. In the report that they published in 1991, they concluded that weight, far from being a contributing factor for cardiovascular disease, seemed to be the opposite. Every eleven-pound increase in body weight was associated with a 10 to 40 percent *lower* chance of having atherosclerosis of the coronary vessels. The fattest people, not the thinnest, had the cleanest arteries. These remarkable findings not only challenge the notion that obesity is a cause of coronary vessel disease, but also suggest the opposite: Obesity may actually be protective!

It must be acknowledged that the one-time-only study cannot give us information about the progress of the disease over time, or which biological or behavioral factors might be associated with the progression, but that limitation does not pertain to the second type of angiographic study. There are similarly provocative findings being issued from some of these surveys. Consider the study conducted by the Cleveland Clinic Foundation, which did two angiographic evaluations of cardiovascular disease in 262 men and women patients, at intervals ranging from two months to fifteen years. If obesity is a cause of vascular heart disease, then the obese patients should be more likely to show evidence of disease progression at their follow-up angiographic evaluations. However, the opposite was the case: A slightly greater percentage of *nonobese* men and women (50 percent *versus* 44 percent) showed evidence of progression.

Just as obesity has been shown to be unrelated to either the presence or the progression of cardiovascular disease, angiographic studies have also shown that weight loss is not a requirement for slowing its progression. The very first study to demonstrate this was published in 1985 in the *New England Journal of Medicine* and was based upon results from the Leiden Intervention Trial in the Netherlands. The thirty-nine subjects in this study, all of whom had atherosclerosis at the beginning of the study, were placed upon a low-fat, vegetarian diet for two years. Though most lost little or no weight, before and after angiograms showed that the progression of the disease had been halted. Dietary intervention had been all that was necessary.

Another fairly recent study to show the benefits of dietary changes, and the irrelevance of obesity, was the Cholesterol Lowering Athero-sclerosis Study done by Dr. David Blankenhorn and his colleagues at the University of Southern California. At the beginning of their two-year study, they weighed and did angiographic evaluations of eighty-two moderately overweight middle-aged men with heart disease (all of whom had had coronary bypass surgery in the past), after which they counseled them about eating a low-fat diet. Two years later they did follow-up weighings and angiograms, and interviewed the men about the extent to which they had followed the dietary advice. Those who had eaten a diet relatively low in fat (averaging 27.5 percent of total calories) showed no new fatty deposits on the walls of their arteries, but the reverse was true for those who had eaten a relatively high-fat diet (averaging 34 percent of total calories). Since neither group had lost weight during the two years, the difference could not be accounted for by total body weight or by changes in body weight. Once again a real measure of improved health had occurred through a dietary change, but one that had nothing to do with weight loss. The authors emphasized that the "appearance of new coronary atherosclerotic lesions can be influenced without weight change by voluntary selection of acceptable foods."

What Ultrasound Tells Us about Obesity and Atherosclerosis

Ultrasound is another biomedical tool that has been used to study cardiovascular disease, and it offers one big advantage over angiography—it is noninvasive, thereby making it easier (certainly for the patient) and less expensive. Several studies have used this technique, which utilizes high-frequency sound waves to determine the degree of atherosclerosis present in arteries, to evaluate the link between vascular disease and the various risk factors considered to play a role. One of the largest involved 15,792 men and women ages 45 to 64—from Minnesota, North Carolina, Maryland, and Mississippi—who volunteered to participate in the Atherosclerosis Risk in Communities (ARIC) Study.

Participants were initially studied between 1987 and 1989, with follow-up measurements every few years through 1998. As might be expected, progression of atherosclerosis over time was significantly linked to smoking, diabetes, and low HDL-cholesterol levels at baseline, and to increases in LDL-cholesterol, triglycerides, and blood pressure during the follow-up years. However, *BMI was not associated with progression of vascular disease over time*—not in men or women, black or white. These findings, published in the January 2002 issue of the *American Journal of Epidemiology*, are similar to those of an earlier, smaller, study of 100 Finnish men.

Although some studies using ultrasound have shown a link between changes in BMI and the progression of this disease over time, the singular importance of a change in BMI is difficult to evaluate—many other variables that could have an impact on both BMI and vascular disease (such as diet and other risk factors, and the fact that in some studies weight loss was induced by surgery) also changed during the course of the study. As mentioned above, the results of the Cholesterol Lowering Atherosclerosis Study indicated that improvements in diet alone, even in the absence of weight loss, could keep atherosclerosis in check.

Atherosclerosis is, of course, only one measure of health—albeit an extremely significant one, given its status as the primary cause of adult mortality in this country. But there are many other risk factors for heart disease, including diabetes, which is a serious disease in and of itself, besides being a risk factor for other diseases; various metabolic disorders, such as insulin resistance and hyperinsulinemia, many of which are part of the diabetic condition; and elevated levels of fat in the blood. They, too, should be looked at for any possible associations with over-weight, weight gain, weight loss, and so forth. There are quite a number of studies that have done just that.

Weight and Its Relationship to Diabetes, Insulin Resistance, Blood-Fat Levels, and Other Risk Factors for Heart Disease

Diabetes is a metabolic disorder afflicting millions of people. Type 2, non-insulin dependent diabetes, also known as adult-onset diabetes because it generally occurs in people over forty, is the most common form of the disease, constituting approximately 90 percent of the diagnosed cases in the United States. Both type 1 and type 2 diabetes are characterized by an impaired ability either to produce or to properly utilize the naturally occurring hormone known as insulin, which is used to metabolize glucose, the body's major source of energy. When the problem is not with insulin production but with the ability to use the insulin effectively, it's known as insulin resistance. (All those with type 2 diabetes are insulin resistant, but not all people with insulin resistance go on to develop diabetes.)

Though both forms of diabetes frequently have a genetic component, individuals with type 2 diabetes can do a great deal to minimize, or even "cure," their condition through proper diet and exercise regimens. Such programs are very effective at dealing with several of the problems caused by insulin resistance—problems that involve not just diabetes, but heart disease, as well. These problems include poor glucose metabolism, high blood pressure, and unhealthy blood-fat profiles, which are characterized by low levels of HDL (the "good" cholesterol) and high levels of LDL (the "bad" cholesterol) and of triglycerides (another form of blood fat).

Since people with type 2 diabetes are very commonly obese, and the diet and exercise programs that frequently help to alleviate their health problems often result in weight loss as well, it has been assumed that obesity itself is a major part of those problems, and weight loss the solution. If weight loss were such a crucial aspect in solving these problems, however, one would expect to see a good correlative relationship between the amount of weight lost and the improvements it is generally thought to be responsible for. Many programs and studies have found that such improvements can come about *when little or even no weight is lost*, as long as certain key changes in activity and diet *are* made.

At the Pritikin Longevity Center in Santa Monica, California, for example, nearly 4,600 people completed their three-week residential program between 1977 and 1988, of whom over 650 had type 2 diabetes. Key features of the program included a high-complex-carbohydrate, high-fiber, low-cholesterol, low-fat, low-salt diet, and lots of daily aerobic exercise, which consisted mainly of walking, about thirty-to-sixty minutes per day. Although many people do lose weight on this program, almost all who start out as obese finish by still being obese, but with one very important difference: greatly improved health.

Of the 652 men and women with type 2 diabetes who completed the three-week program, 71 percent of those who had been taking oral hypoglycemic drugs to increase insulin production were able to go off their medications; 76 percent of those who were not taking medication had reduced their blood glucose to normal levels; and 39 percent of those taking insulin were able to discontinue it. For all patients combined, total cholesterol, LDL cholesterol, and triglycerides were reduced by 21 to 38 percent; blood pressures by about 7 to 15 percent. Close to 80 percent of the hypertensives in the program were able to reduce their blood pressure and discontinue taking the hypertension drugs. This is a particularly heartening finding, since many of these drugs, for example the diuretics and the beta blockers, can cause metabolic problems such as insulin resistance—a major factor in both heart disease and type 2 diabetes. The current thinking is that some 350,000 cases of type 2 diabetes may be attributable to doctor-prescribed drugs.

Since most participants in the Pritikin Program did shed some pounds during the three weeks, it might seem logical to conclude that weight loss itself played a pivotal role in the health improvements. A closer look at the results suggests that this is not the case. Consider total cholesterol, which decreased from 234 mg/dl to 181 mg/dl, and LDL cholesterol, which decreased from 152 mg/dl to 117 mg/dl. These are very impressive improvements, and, it should be noted, rival those of many cholesterol-lowering medications. However, statistical analysis of the data revealed that 99.5 percent of the decreases in both types of cholesterol were attributable to factors *other than weight loss.* Similarly, obesity itself appeared to play a relatively unimportant role in the participants' problems with insulin, as emphasized by the authors: "Thus, it appears that obesity itself does not create insulin resistance because many of the subjects in the present study had normalized their insulin levels, but were still significantly overweight or obese at the end of the program." The authors went on to say that their data suggest that "attention should be focused more on the quality of food consumed as opposed to the quantity of food and weight loss *per se.*"

Are the Pritikin Program results an anomaly? No, they can happen anywhere. Diet and exercise, alone or in combination, are far more important than weight, or weight loss, in improving the health of persons either with diabetes or heart disease, or of those who have risk factors for these diseases. The following examples illustrate:

- In the Dietary Approaches to Stop Hypertension (DASH) clinical trial, 459 overweight men and women were assigned to either a control (typical American) diet or to one of two dietary change groups. One hundred thirty-three of the participants had high blood pressure. One of these groups was encouraged to just eat more fruits and vegetables; the other was encouraged to eat more fruits and vegetables, and also to consume more low-fat dairy products and less total fat (the "combination" diet). The study lasted eight weeks, and food intake was controlled so that each person's weight did not change. Among 133 subjects with hypertension, those on the combination diet reduced both systolic and diastolic blood pressures significantly, by a little over 11 mmHg and 5 mmHg, respectively. In the report, published in the April 17, 1997, issue of the *New England Journal of Medicine*, the authors underscored the fact that blood pressures in moderately hypertensive, overweight men and women could be reduced without weight loss, and, it should be emphasized, by an amount similar in magnitude to that observed with antihypertensive medications.

• Researchers at National Public Health Institute, in Helsinki, evaluated the effects of diet on cholesterol levels of 54 men and women who had high cholesterol levels to begin with. The subjects consumed a relatively low-fat (24 percent of total calories) diet for a period of six weeks, and then switched back to their habitual diet, very high in fat (39 percent of total calories). For the 24 women in the study total cholesterol decreased from 239 mg/dl to 188 mg/dl during the low-fat diet period (similar to the Pritikin results), and then went right back up to 231 mg/dl when they returned to their regular diet. For the men total cholesterol decreased from 263 mg/dl to 201 mg/dl during the low-fat diet period, and shot back up to 259 mg/dl when they switched back to their normal diet. Although body weights decreased by an average of a couple pounds on the low-fat diet, body weight did not change at all during the 6-week period in which they returned to their normal diet. The researchers highlighted the significance of this in their conclusions, published in the September 30, 1982, issue of the *New England Journal of Medicine*: "Despite the constant body weight, the serum lipids and lipoproteins returned to their original levels, indicating that the observed changes were due to the composition of the diet and not to the reduction in weight."

• At Laval University, in Quebec, Canada, 31 obese women completed a 6-month aerobic exercise program, consisting of moderate aerobic exercise 4 to 5 days per week. As expected, most of the women lost body fat—an average of about 6 pounds. Interestingly, 11 of the 31 women actually *gained* body fat during the program, with the average gain about 6 pounds (which suggests that these "gainers" may have overcompensated during the study by consuming more calories each day than their bodies needed, in order to replace those burned off during the exercise). Nevertheless, both losers *and gainers* improved cardiovascular fitness by the same amount. Furthermore, the women who gained body fat also improved their insulin sensitivity by the same amount as the women who lost weight. Improvements in total cholesterol and HDL cholesterol were also similar, suggesting that it was the exercise, and not the fat loss, that was the key to health and fitness improvements.

I could go on and on. The point is: *It is possible to greatly improve or even "cure" diabetes and other serious health problems, such as high blood pressure and elevated blood fats, while remaining markedly overweight or obese.*

If we were to extrapolate from the results achieved by the Pritikin Program and all of the other studies with similar findings, the potential health implications could be staggering. There are an estimated 16 million people with type 2 diabetes in the United States, perhaps another 50 million insulin-resistant people who have undiagnosed problems with glucose metabolism (which may or may not eventually develop into diabetes), and approximately 58 million hypertensives. Putting the entire country on a nutrition and exercise regimen similar to those described would mean that something like 12 million diabetics, 46 million hypertensives, and at least 35 million insulin-resistant individuals could be "cured" or greatly improved within a month or so. Weight loss would have little, if anything, to do with it.

We now know that most obese people can normalize such disorders as high blood pressure, high blood fats, and insulin resistance, *while remaining obese.* Chances are they will be healthier if they stay that way; trying to conform to any arbitrary height-weight standards, especially by dieting, may harm their health. For example, weight loss that is achieved by many of the fad diets of the past few decades, especially the low-carbohydrate and relatively high-fat ones, can greatly increase the risk of heart disease. This may explain in part why those who diet to lose weight—typically people with heavier-than-average BMIs—have been shown to have higher rates for heart disease, high blood pressure, and type 2 diabetes than those who never diet. This latter observation may in turn help to expose the faulty logic behind the present-day attempts to *quantify* the annual "body count" attributed to obesity.

Obesity Allegedly Kills 300,000 Americans Every Year: Where Is the Evidence?

When the chair of the scientific panel at the 1985 NIH conference on obesity asserted that "obesity is a killer," he did not quantify the death toll attributed to excess body fat. That would come nearly a decade later, when former surgeon general C. Everett Koop, in launching his "Shape Up America" campaign in a White House ceremony presided over by former first Lady Hillary Rodham Clinton, claimed that obesity kills 300,000 Americans every year.

Subsequently, this statistic has surfaced repeatedly in newspapers, magazines, television and radio broadcasts, and in many scientific and medical journals—each time proclaiming obesity the second leading preventable cause of death (next to smoking) in the United States. Cited at the 1995 Food and Drug Administration (FDA) hearings on dexfenfluramine (Redux), this ominous statistic was perhaps the single most compelling reason for that ill-fated weight-loss drug's approval (Redux was removed from the market in 1997 due to health risks). In an editorial published in the August 29, 1996, issue of the *New England Journal of Medicine,* two physicians—Dr. JoAnn Manson, from Harvard Medical School, and Dr. Gerald Reich, from the University of Pennsylvania—argued that "Obesity is the second leading cause of preventable death in the United States...and it contributes to 300,000 deaths annually." In the December 18, 1996, issue of the *Journal of the American Medical Association*, the National Task Force on the Prevention and Treatment of Obesity declared, "Obesity-related conditions are estimated to contribute to 300,000 deaths yearly." In January 1997, the American Dietetic Association, in its position paper on weight management published in its own journal, maintained, "Obesity-related medical conditions are the second leading cause of preventable death in America, resulting in 300,000 lives lost each year." Later that year, in a letter to the editor appearing in the May 12, 1997 issue of *Newsweek* (in response to an April 21 dogma-challenging cover story entitled, "Does It Matter What You Weigh?"), Linda Webb Carilli, general manager of corporate affairs for Weight Watchers International, wrote, "Obesity costs the nation more than $100 billion annually, and causes the premature deaths of approximately 300,000 people each year."

What surprises me, given the gravity of the statistic, is that no one seems to have bothered to verify it. Then again, perhaps the indoctrination about the evils of body fat has been so thorough that the unquestioned acceptance of the obesity body count is understandable. At the kick-off for Shape Up America, for example, Dr. Koop provided no source for the "obesity kills" statistic. Also, when questioned by a reporter from the *Wall Street Journal* at the peak of the fen-phen debacle, in September 1997, James Bilstad, director of the FDA's office for drug evaluation and the person who made the final decision to approve Redux, stated that he was unaware of the source of the statistic— despite the fact that the 300,000 "death toll" from obesity was instrumental in the drug's approval.

Several published reports, however, including those mentioned above, did cite one source for the statistic—a paper entitled, "Actual Causes of Death in the United States," published in the November 10, 1993 issue of the *Journal of the American Medical Association*. But a close examination of this paper, written by Drs. J Michael McGinnis (at the time Deputy Assistant Secretary for Health, Disease Prevention and Health Promotion) and William H. Foege, of Emory University, reveals no such assertions about obesity. Drs. McGinnis and Foege had analyzed all the relevant epidemiological research and provided estimates of the number of deaths that could be attributed to various "contributing causes." Number one on the list, at 400,000 deaths per year, was tobacco. Number two on the list, at 300,000 deaths per year, was "diet/activity patterns." Obesity itself did not even appear on their list.

Although it's quite evident that a junk-food diet and couch potato lifestyle can lead to obesity, it is absolutely unjustifiable to equate behavioral patterns (poor diet and physical inactivity, in this instance) with a physical characteristic (obesity). Even so, that is apparently, and unfortunately, what happened. Countless studies show that poor diet and a sedentary lifestyle adversely affect the health of individuals across the entire weight spectrum, not just fat people. Therefore, use of this statistic to support the assertion that obesity *itself* kills 300,000 Americans every year is without merit. Drs. McGinnis and Foege attempted to correct the persistent misuse of their cause-of-death estimates when, in 1998, they wrote in the *New England Journal of Medicine*, "The figure applies broadly to the combined effects of various dietary factors and activity patterns that are too sedentary, not to the narrower effect of obesity alone. Indeed, given the contribution of multiple diet-related factors to problems such as high blood pressure, heart disease, and cancer, we noted explicitly the difficulty of sorting out the independent contribution of any one factor."

A New Source for the 300,000 Figure—But Still No Evidence

Yet the statistic lives on. For example, in the 2001 "Surgeon General's Call to Action to Prevent and Decrease Overweight and Obesity," Dr. David Satcher, surgeon general at the time, stated in his foreword to the report, "Approximately 300,000 deaths each year in this country are currently associated with overweight and obesity." (Interestingly— and rather inexplicably—the report itself actually states otherwise: "Unhealthy dietary habits and sedentary behavior together account for approximately 300,000 deaths every year." Nevertheless it's plainly evident that obesity, not "diet/activity patterns," is viewed as the real health problem, as this statement appears in the opening section entitled "Overweight and Obesity as Public Health Problems in America.") Although the 300,000 figure is still the same, a new source is now cited: "Annual Deaths Attributable to Obesity in the United States," published in the October 27, 1999, issue of the *Journal of the American Medical Association*. Based on their analysis of data from six epidemiological studies, the authors of the report concluded that "obesity is a major cause of mortality in the United States," accounting for approximately 300,000 deaths each year. A closer scrutiny of the logic behind their calculations, however, suggests that the authors of this report, who were led by David Allison of Columbia University College of Physicians and Surgeons, in New York, greatly overstated their conclusion.

To estimate the annual number of deaths attributable to obesity, Dr. Allison and his colleagues first calculated "hazard ratios" (death risks) for all the various BMI groupings in the six studies selected (which included the Framingham Heart Study, Nurses' Health Study, Tecumseh Community Health Study, Alameda Community Health Study, American Cancer Society Prevention Study I, and the National Health and Nutrition Examination Survey I Epidemiologic Follow-up Study). In general, hazard ratios increased as BMI increased beyond about 25 to 27; for example, men and women with BMIs between 30 and 35 had a roughly 50 percent higher death risk, compared to men and women with BMIs between 23 and 25. (It must be noted that a number of additional epidemiological studies of BMI and mortality—not evaluated by the authors of this report—show a quite different picture for BMI and death risk, as will be discussed in the next chapter.) Then, by using three additional pieces of information—the size of the U.S. adult population; the number of men and women in each BMI category; and the total annual number of deaths in the country—hazard ratios were converted to actual numbers of deaths by extrapolation from each of the six studies to the entire U.S. population. Depending upon the study, annual death toll estimates attributable to obesity ranged from 236,111 to 383,410, with an overall average of approximately 300,000. Hence the authors' conclusion that obesity is a "major cause of mortality in the United States."

Hold on. As the saying goes, there are three kinds of lies, and one of them is statistics. In reading this paper, and many previous papers written by the authors of this report, it is apparent that the investigators designed their statistical analysis with preconceived—and very much mainstream—notions about obesity and health. To arrive at their conclusions, they may have used statistics "as a drunken man uses a lamppost, more for support than illumination."

The fatal flaw in their analysis is best revealed by the authors' own admission: "Our calculations assume that all (controlling for age, sex, and smoking) excess mortality in obese people is due to their adiposity." Thus the authors made no attempt to determine whether other factors—

such as physical inactivity, low fitness levels, poor diet, risky weight-loss practices, and less than adequate access to health care, just to name a few—could have explained some, or all, of the excess mortality in fat people.

Overweight and obese individuals are more likely to be sedentary and have lower aerobic fitness levels than nonoverweight persons are. Both sedentary lifestyle and low aerobic fitness (which can be altered independently of weight loss) greatly increase the risk of premature death. So it's entirely possible that much of the health risk associated with obesity is really due to a lack of exercise and associated low fitness levels. In fact, data from the Aerobics Center Longitudinal Study, in Dallas, Texas (to be discussed in detail in the next chapter), show that low aerobic fitness levels account for 100 percent of the excess mortality among obese men (that is, aerobically-fit, fat men have death rates no higher than their thinner counterparts). Had Dr. Allison and colleagues used the fat-and-fit men from the Aerobic Center Longitudinal Study in their calculations, the annual death toll attributable to obesity would be essentially zero! (Low fitness, on the other hand, would be tagged as the "major cause of mortality.")

Low fitness and sedentary lifestyle, however, aren't the only factors that might explain the higher mortality rates of obese persons. The prevalence of dieting, particularly yo-yo dieting, is much greater among obese people, especially women. Consequently, obese people are far more likely to experience extreme weight fluctuations during their lifetime. As mentioned earlier in this chapter, weight cycling may increase the risk of high blood pressure. Weight cycling also has been reported to increase the risk of premature death (which will be discussed in detail in Chapter 7). A 1991 report from the Framingham Heart Study (which is one of the studies used by Dr. Allison and colleagues to generate the "obesity kills" statistic) revealed that virtually all of the "excess" cardio-vascular disease mortality in obese men and women could be explained by lifetime weight fluctuation.

Obese women and men are also far more likely to have tried extreme, and calorically unbalanced, diets, such as starvation-type fasting and liquid protein diets. Although these practices are less common today, they were very popular in recent past decades (for example, the 1950s, 1960s, and 1970s)—during which time most of the epidemiological studies of BMI and mortality (including the six used by Dr. Allison and colleagues) had been initiated. Also, obese women and men are considerably more likely to take weight-loss drugs. Although this will be explored more in Chapter 7, it is necessary to mention for the sake of the present discussion that many of the weight-loss drugs that have been used over the years have serious, sometimes fatal, consequences.

I could go on. My point is that no published report on the alleged annual death toll attributable to obesity has satisfactorily eliminated the possibility that the higher death rates observed in women and men with higher-than-average BMIs are instead caused by one or more of the many possible contributing factors, such as those mentioned above, that are more prevalent in this population. Until that happens, the "obesity kills" hypothesis remains just that—a hypothesis. As Dr. Elizabeth Barrett-Conner pointed out in her testimony at the 1985 NIH conference on obesity, it's one that, even 17 years after she spoke, "the available data do not support."

It appears that thinness, rather than obesity, may be a risk factor in many diseases. Though this may be just another variation on the kind of guilt-by-association case that has been made against obesity, it's an interesting and little-explored hypothesis. We'll look at the evidence for and against thinness, and more generally for and against any measure of weight as a risk factor in any disease, in the next chapter.

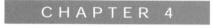

CHAPTER 4

Thinner May Not
Be Healthier

We have, in effect, an Eleventh Commandment. We have come to believe thinner is healthier, happier, and more beautiful as though it were handed down on Mount Sinai. But these are not divine truths—they are prejudices with a complex history. They have led to a false religion that does not deliver what it promises.

—Roberta Pollack Seid, *Never Too Thin:*
Why Women Are at War with Their Bodies

To see the false religion of thinness at work, let's consider our reaction to a hypothetical case—that of a nonsmoking, middle-aged man who has a heart attack while sitting quietly, watching television. Over the years his blood pressure and cholesterol level have been a little on the high side, but within the normal range. However, at 5'10", with a medium frame, he happens to weigh 195 pounds, which is about 24 percent over the midpoint of what is recommended for his height by the Met Life height-weight tables (151-163). He also has a BMI of 28—overweight by two different sets of medical standards. Why did he suffer the heart attack? Though there are a number of plausible answers, most people presented with this scenario, including those in the medical and life insurance industries, would be inclined to blame his heart attack on his weight— a conclusion they have been led to by the ubiquitous height-weight tables and the proselytizing that accompanies them. After all, just about all of our major diseases *have* been blamed on "overweight." The belief that thin people live healthier and longer lives than heavy people is so deeply rooted in our culture and medical mind-set that it is seldom questioned.

Of all our convictions about health, "thinner is healthier" has no rival when it comes to the gap between belief and evidence. There is a lot of evidence that suggests the opposite, evidence that has for the most part gone unheeded, never having made the leap from medical journals into the popular press. But if we do go to the medical and scientific journals, we discover many studies suggesting that thinness does not guarantee good health or greater longevity, and losing weight does not necessarily make us healthier. In fact, the reverse may be true. Extra pounds do not inevitably carry with them the likelihood of poor health or an early demise, and may, for some diseases, be an advantage, both in incidence rates and in mortality rates. Being overweight is a problem only when we exceed "natural," as opposed to arbitrarily defined, culturally and medically imposed weight ranges.

Natural Weights

Each of us has a "natural" weight, which we will not find on any height-weight chart. The simplest way of defining that weight is to say that it is the weight at which the body feels healthy and is healthy, and is free of the risk factors that are within our control for such major killers as heart and artery disease, diabetes, and cancer. Those who are naturally meant to be heavier than culturally or medically imposed standards are healthier when they are heavier; those who are naturally meant to be thinner than those standards are better off thinner; and those whom nature intended to be about average weight are better off at about average weight. From this perspective, weight as a yardstick of health ceases to have any validity, with the exception of the relatively few at the far extremes—the markedly emaciated and the extremely obese. (Although more than one-half of U.S. adults are considered overweight or obese by BMI criteria, only three percent of men and women in America have BMIs greater than 40, which is classified as "extremely obese." Between two and three percent are considered underweight.)

The discrepancy between the popular conviction and this much more skeptical view of weight as a meaningful measure has to do with *causality*, which is next to impossible to establish in large population-based studies. When, as is often the case, overweight is *associated with* health problems, that may well be because the same behaviors that resulted in the problems also resulted in the excess poundage. Look again at the man who suffered the heart attack. It could be that his weight is a natural weight for him, which in no way contributed to his heart attack, but that he had a strong genetic predisposition to heart disease, as indicated by the fact that his father and mother both died of heart attacks in their fifties, despite being at recommended weights. It could also be the case that his weight was no problem, but he had just lost his job in a management shake-up and was worried about how to pay college tuition for his three teenagers—stress being a known risk factor for heart attacks. However, if he was over his natural weight, it is likely that he, like most middle-aged American males, put on his excess weight as a result of exercising too little, and consuming a diet too high in fat and sugar and too low in fiber. Both of these behaviors greatly increase the risk for heart disease and also cause weight gain. This last scenario suggests that his excess weight may be nothing more than the visible, but relatively benign, consequence of a sedentary lifestyle and poor dietary habits.

Fat and Fit

One way to put this hypothesis to the test is to find a group of people who weigh a lot for their height, but who also happen to be very physically fit (as measured by standard stress and endurance tests), and to track them over time to see whether they're healthy (as measured by their rate of premature mortality). This is not hard to do, for a fair number of men and women falls into the overweight-but-fit description, as Dr. Steven Blair and his associates at the Cooper Institute for Aerobics Research in Dallas, Texas, found out. Since 1970 Dr. Blair and his research team have enrolled more than 26,000 men and more than 8,000 women in the Aerobics Center Longitudinal Study to assess the possible role of physical fitness in reducing mortality rates. Their subjects varied in age from twenty to ninety, and were admitted into the study only if they seemed to be in good health on the basis of a number of different diagnostic tests. Once admitted to the study, which is still going on, the subjects underwent a battery of additional health and fitness tests at the institute. Although the primary purpose is to study the possible benefits of physical fitness, the role of body weight has also been considered. In one of their first reports, issued in 1989 and covering results through 1985, the researchers found that, contrary to conventional wisdom, being heavy did not increase the risk of dying prematurely. When considered in combination with fitness level, being overweight seemed to be better than being underweight.

For example, a 5'10", physically fit, middle-aged man was nearly twice as likely to die prematurely if he weighed 138 pounds or less as opposed to weighing 175 pounds or more. The same result was observed for women. A 5'4", physically fit, middle-aged woman had almost half the risk of premature death at 146 pounds or more as at 115 pounds or less, though the 115 weight fell within Met Life's guidelines for recommended weight in both 1959 and 1983. However, fitness, not weight, was the factor that mattered most. Dr. Blair found that the least fit overweight men and women had more than twice the risk of premature death as did the fittest overweight men and women. Other figures in the study reinforced the importance of fitness.

One of the drawbacks of this initial report was that no information was provided on the actual body composition of the subjects. A skeptic could argue that the excess weight on the bodies of overweight-but-fit men and women was muscle, not fat. If so, it would imply that the combination of being fit and having a lot of muscle mass is a good thing, a scenario wholly compatible with conventional wisdom.

However, a more recent report from these researchers undermined this conventional wisdom and actually strengthened the fat-and-fit hypothesis. This time the researchers focused their attention just on the 21,925 men who had body composition assessments in addition to fitness tests. Men were classified as lean (body fat less than 16.7 percent of total body weight), normal (body fat between 16.7 percent and 25.0 percent), or obese (greater than 25 percent body fat), and as either fit or unfit—thus allowing for six different categories based on fitness and body composition. Fitness was defined in terms of how long it took each man to reach fatigue during a treadmill exercise test. To be considered "fit" a man only needed to be in the top 80 percent of his age group—a rather generous definition of "fit." For example, this level of fitness could be achieved by taking a brisk walk, at about 3 to 4 miles per hour, for approximately 30 minutes, four or five days per week. The results confirmed the "fat and fit" hypothesis—and also provided a few other surprising findings.

Obese-fit men had death rates that were just as low as lean-fit men, and, perhaps more importantly, had death rates that were one-half that of lean-unfit men—indicating that fitness is more important than leanness in terms of avoiding premature death. The results were the same whether body fatness was expressed as a percentage of total weight or in terms of actual pounds of body fat. For example, a fit man carrying 50 pounds of body fat had a death rate less than one-half that of an unfit man with only 25 pounds of body fat. Fitness mattered, fatness did not. Neither did leanness, as demonstrated by the somewhat surprising finding that fat-free body mass provided no protection against early mortality. Fat-free, or lean body, mass is the sum of all body tissues other than fat; most fat-free mass is muscle. The highest death rates were observed in unfit men with high amounts of fat-free mass (perhaps former athletes-turned-couch potatoes). By contrast the lowest death rates were observed in fit men with low amounts of fat-free mass. Since muscularity correlates fairly well with fat-free mass, this strongly suggests that merely having a large muscle mass is no guarantee of good health. Data on women enrolled in the Aerobics Center Longitudinal Study also support the fat-and-fit hypothesis.

Since Dr. Blair's study did not measure each person's body weight change over time, we cannot use it to assess another belief current in the anti-obesity establishment—that gaining weight after one's twenties increases one's chance of premature death. From the 1942 Met Life weight tables, which eliminated age as a variable, down to the September 12, 2001, issue of the *Journal of the American Medical Association*, in which some of the latest findings from the annual Behavioral Risk Factor Surveillance System survey were presented, the message is that while it may be normal to gain weight with age, it certainly isn't healthy.

But a study that has been going on for the past four decades suggests quite the opposite—that weight gain over time may be not only normal, but healthy, too. Dr. Ralph Paffenbarger, now-professor emeritus in the Department of Family, Community and Preventive Medicine at Stanford University, has been tracking the health and mortality facts pertaining to nearly seventeen thousand Harvard alumni who had entered the university between the years 1916 and 1950. Only those alumni who had no diagnosed health problems at the time Dr. Paffenbarger and his research team initially contacted them, early in the 1960s, were accepted into the program.

At the beginning of the study all the alumni, who were roughly between the ages of thirty and sixty-five, were asked to fill out questionnaires on attributes and behaviors thought to have a potential impact on health. These included body weight and physical activity, which was categorized according to calories expended, from less than 500 per week to more than 2,000. As the men died during the years of follow-up, the causes of death were reported and attempts made to correlate various risk factors to mortality rates.

The men who had the best chance of living a long life were those who gained the most weight (as expressed in BMI units) since their college days *who also expended at least 2,000 calories per week in physical activities such as walking, climbing stairs, and playing in various sports.* The amount of weight gained by these men was not trivial—about twenty-five pounds or more for most of them. Depending on the level of physical activity, men who gained more than about twenty-five pounds since college had a 19 to 32 percent lower mortality rate than men who gained less than about fifteen pounds. This should not be taken as a recommendation to pack on more pounds as you get older, for the weight gain cannot be considered independent of the effects of the physical activity. Those who gained at least fifteen pounds or more since college but were very sedentary had mortality rates that were 53 to 96 percent higher than men who had gained a similar amount of weight but were physically active. Clearly weight and weight gain by themselves provide little meaningful information about health. Only when they are viewed in the context of the lifestyle that helped to produce the weight can their impact—or lack of impact—be assessed.

Despite the fact that these landmark studies were published in major medical and scientific journals (Blair's in the *Journal of the American Medical Association* in 1989 and in the *American Journal of Clinical Nutrition* in 1999; and Paffenbarger's in the *New England Journal of Medicine* in 1986), their findings about weight and mortality have gone largely ignored. The emphasis in all the reporting has been on the positive impact of physical exercise, which is all to the good. But better still would be an acknowledgment that weight itself does not appear to be as important a risk factor for premature mortality as is commonly believed. The results of these studies demonstrate that unless the facts about physical fitness and activity are plugged into the complex and still incompletely understood equation that determines well-being, we can say very little of any significance about the impact of weight on health.

Other factors that influence health, such as nutrition, dieting behavior, weight fluctuation, and stress, must also be considered, but to mention these is just to scratch the surface. Scores of factors that have a potential impact on health, positive as well as negative, have been uncovered by researchers. For heart disease alone, at least 246 separate risk factors have been postulated as causal or contributing agents. Designing a study to separate out any one factor as causal, whether it is weight or any of the other 245 possibilities, is an extraordinarily difficult, if not impossible, thing to do. As of 2002 there has not been a single study that has truly evaluated the effects of weight alone on health, which means that "thinner is healthier" is not a fact, but an unsubstantiated hypothesis for which there is a wealth of evidence that suggests the reverse.

Why, then, has the "thinner is healthier" creed been handed down from one generation to the next as though it had originated from Moses? To fully understand how this happened, it is necessary to take a closer look at the life insurance studies on which it is based, and the impact these studies have had on the scientific mind-set since the 1950s, despite the fact that they had extremely serious flaws over and above the failure to consider weight in combination with other factors as a health risk.

Analyzing the Actuarial Data

The two biggest studies were the 1959 Build and Blood Pressure Study, which covered people who bought life insurance policies between the years 1935 and 1954, and the 1979 Build Study, which covered people who bought policies between the years 1954 and 1972. Demographically, life insurance policyholders are not representative of America as a whole, of course. Aside from economic, racial, and ethnic factors that would make them a nonrepresentative cross-section, they tended to weigh between five and ten pounds less than the average American and, perhaps in part because the insurance companies had been successful in screening out bad risks, to have mortality rates up to 40 percent lower than the general population.

However, the demographic problems are insignificant compared with the flaws in the methodology of the mortality-risk-factor assessment— beginning with the very definition of *mortality*. The insurance companies defined mortality as the cashing in of a policy, not the death of a person. If a man had purchased three policies and subsequently died, his death would count as three deaths. In the 1959 study this meant that there were nearly one-fifth more "policy deaths" than policyholders who actually died. How this quirky bit of data management may have skewed the figures it is impossible to say. But there is no doubt that any well-designed scientific study would not allow this sort of sample-size embellishment.

The life insurance studies also fall short of accepted scientific standards by their failure to define a population database. That is, they do not measure a fixed, unchanging population sample. Anybody who bought a policy during the years of the studies was included. So, regardless of whether a person bought a policy in 1935 or in 1953, he or she was included in the 1959 study. So, although it sounds impressive on the basis of number of people being assessed and the period of time being covered, the average follow-up for what sounds like a 20-year study was actually *only 7.8 years.*

Another major problem with the actuarial data stems from the fact that the life insurance companies knew virtually nothing about the lifestyles of the policyholders. Though their weights were always recorded, applicants for policies were never questioned about their eating or exercise habits. The reliance on weight as the most important indicator of health risk had begun in the early 1900s, when weight was the easiest variable to measure, and little was known about other potential risk factors or how to measure them.

As far as the insurance companies are concerned, weight has remained the key variable ever since, which is not to say that the insurance companies' studies have been rigorous even in their reporting or in their analysis of that one key variable. Roughly 10 to 20 percent of the weights and heights used in the actuarial data were self-reported, a methodology sure to result in inaccuracies. Even more problematic is the fact that the insurance companies recorded each policyholder's weight only once, at the time of the application for insurance, and then never again. Nothing was known about overall weight gain or loss over time, or about weight fluctuation.

How such limited information might influence the interpretation of the actuarial data is illustrated by the following hypothetical case. Two 5'4", forty-year-old nonsmoking women, buy life insurance at the same time. One weighs 130 pounds at the time she purchases her policy, gains 30 pounds over the next fifteen years—meaning she is clinically overweight by BMI standards—and is still alive when the study is over. The other weighs 160 pounds at the time she buys insurance, and chronically diets to lose weight. After fifteen years she dies of a heart attack shortly after losing 30 pounds on a crash diet. While it would be merely speculative to conclude that gaining 30 pounds did the first woman any good, or that losing 30 pounds on a crash diet after years of chronic weight fluctuation did the second woman any harm, surely it is equally speculative to conclude that the one piece of actuarial data recorded by the studies—weight at time of policy purchase—has any meaning. Nonetheless the studies did reach a conclusion, which was not presented as speculative: 130 pounds is a good weight for a five-foot-four-inch woman, 160 pounds is a bad weight.

This "conclusion" is at odds, of course, with the actual weight and mortality experiences of our two hypothetical women; and, given the weight fluctuation typical of the U.S. population, may have been at odds with the experiences of most of the insured. Over one sample ten-year period, the CDC found that approximately three-fourths of adult Americans gained or lost the equivalent of 5 percent or more of their body weight, and more than one-half of the adults experienced weight changes of up to 15 percent of their body weight. If we assume that policyholders were anything like those surveyed by the CDC, we realize that by virtue of the fact that only one weight was recorded for each policyholder, the actuarial data cannot tell us much, if anything, about the impact of weight on health.

All these study flaws notwithstanding, the life insurance industry's conclusions have been accepted widely, if not quite universally, as biological truth. Though similar flaws marred the results of all the preceding life insurance studies as well, there have been but a few lone voices in the medical and scientific communities speaking up about the need to critically evaluate the data. As a result, the unwarranted assumption that weight is a primary determinant of health problems was officially embraced by the medical establishment in 1951 (when the AMA and the U.S. Public Health Service joined Met Life in its antiobesity crusade) and has been dominating and contaminating scientific investigations of the impact of weight on mortality ever since. Not only do researchers tend to begin their studies without the open mind that is the hallmark of an impartial investigative process, but the design of their studies often duplicates many of the shortcomings of the actuarial studies.

Consider, for example, the Nurses' Health Study, which has been scaring people with its alarming conclusions about the health risks of gaining weight ever since its two front-page news-making scientific reports were released in 1995. Sponsored by the NIH, researchers at Brigham and Women's Hospital in Boston have been tracking over 115,000 married female nurses in eleven different states since 1976, mailing them questionnaires every two years to keep track of deaths and of newly diagnosed cases of serious illness. The nurses, who were thirty to fifty-five at the time the study began, were asked how much they weighed at time of entry to the study, and how much they estimated they had weighed at age eighteen. Compared to those who had gained—or lost—less than about 10 pounds since age 18, those who gained more than this amount of weight in most instances had a higher risk of coronary heart disease.

The results for modest weight gain, however, were inconsistent. For example, in the February 8, 1995, issue of *JAMA*, the Nurses' Health Study researchers reported that a weight gain of eleven to seventeen pounds since age eighteen was associated with a 25 percent higher risk of coronary heart disease. Later that year, on the other hand, the researchers reported in the September 14 issue of the *New England Journal of Medicine* that a weight gain of up to twenty pounds after the age of eighteen did not increase the risk of dying from coronary heart disease. In fact, the risk associated with this degree of weight gain was 30 percent *lower* compared to women who had remained fairly weight stable (although this was not statistically significant). The researchers offered no explanation for the inconsistent findings.

What is interesting about the design of this study is that not only did it not appropriately take into account behavioral factors such as exercise and dieting, but it *refused* to acknowledge possible risk factors such as high blood pressure, low HDL and high LDL cholesterol, high levels of triglycerides, and high insulin levels. Though many researchers believe these risk factors to be the results of the same unhealthy behaviors that result in overweight (dietary intake that is high in fat and sugar, and low in fiber; a sedentary lifestyle), with weight being, for the most part, a neutral side effect, the Nurses' Health Study researchers believe the reverse: Overweight itself *causes* those risk factors. On that assumption their results were almost a foregone conclusion. Interestingly enough, however, this same study's results concerning the incidence of breast cancer told a very different story about weight as a risk factor, as will be discussed later in the chapter.

Framingham Heart Study —1983 Report

Another study much cited in the antiobesity camp is the Framingham Heart Study, which began in 1948 and is still going on today, making it the longest-running major epidemiological study in the United States. Commissioned by the NIH for the purpose of studying risk factors for cardiovascular disease, it had a population database of 5,209 men and women between the ages of twenty-eight and sixty-two, who all lived in the community of Framingham, Massachusetts. Over the years, this study has issued a series of reports on its findings, one of the most influential of which was the one published in 1983 in *Circulation*, the flagship journal of the American Heart Association. Under the title "Obesity as an Independent Risk Factor for Cardiovascular Disease: A 26-Year Follow-up of Participants in the Framingham Heart Study," it made what sounded like a convincing case for the standard conclusions: Being overweight, and gaining weight after the age of twenty-five, dramatically increased the risk of developing cardiovascular disease.

In an improvement over the life insurance studies, it did consider and its statistics were designed to take into account such independent variables as cholesterol levels, blood pressure, and smoking. However, as with the life insurance studies, there was no attempt to consider exercise, physical fitness, diet, stress, or other variables and risk factors that we now understand to be of potential significance. Even more problematic, given the conclusion it drew about weight gain after twenty-five, is the fact that the study did not incorporate data in regard to weight change over time. Though weight was measured every two years, those measurements were not analyzed for purposes of the study. Instead the only measurements the researchers used were the subjects' weight at the time the study began, and the weight the subjects estimated themselves to have been at age twenty-five. As a result, it is impossible for this study to draw scientifically valid conclusions about weight gain, or about weight itself.

How the results might have differed if the study had been better designed—had it, for example, taken exercise into account—is suggested by a subsequent report from the Heart Study, in 1989, which was based on findings about the children of the original Framingham participants. Ranging in age from twenty to sixty-nine, the 3,360 subjects of this later study were surveyed about their exercise habits, thus enabling the researchers to draw positive connections between higher levels of exercise and healthier levels of HDL cholesterol and triglycerides in the blood *as well as* lower weights. Most of the thin people exercised more and had better blood profiles than most of the fat people. Since blood-fat measurements are considered key to an assessment of cardiovascular risk, and it is well documented that exercise can affect these measurements in a beneficial manner, it is entirely possible that the "overweight" men and women of the earlier Framingham report experienced their increased cardiovascular mortality rates because of the consequences of physical inactivity, with overweight being a relatively harmless side effect of that inactivity, as Drs. Blair and Paffenbarger observed in their studies. Nonetheless the 1983 paper continues to be cited as definitive proof of the negative effect of obesity on health.

Framingham Heart Study —1991 Report

Interestingly enough, a later report on the original Framingham subjects, issued in 1991 under the title "Variability of Body Weight and

Health Outcomes in the Framingham Population," also undermines some of the conclusions of the 1983 report, particularly as they pertain to weight gain. This study had an additional six years of follow-up for a total of thirty-two, and did incorporate the data concerning the biannual weight measurements that were taken, thus enabling the researchers to see characteristic patterns of weight change for each participant—stability, steady gain or steady loss, or chronic fluctuation. Their goal was to study the effects of weight change on the risk of developing either coronary heart disease or cancer, and on the risk of dying either from heart disease, or from any and all causes. Weight gain was associated with a significantly lower risk of *developing* heart disease in men, and of *dying* from heart disease in both men and women. Weight gain also decreased overall mortality rates in both men and women.

So when you put the 1983 and the 1991 studies together, this is the picture you get: Weight gain from age twenty-five to time of entry into the study (which participants were asked to estimate) is bad from the standpoint of developing heart trouble. But once a person gains the weight, his or her chances of dying—not only from heart disease but from all causes—are lower if the weight is either maintained or increased, and higher if weight is lost. In addition, a high average BMI did not significantly increase total mortality in either men or women, nor did it increase the risk of developing cancer. (More about the Framingham study and cancer below.) Going against so much of the prevailing wisdom about overweight, weight gain, weight loss, and weight fluctuation, this study was seen as confusing and inconclusive, as compared to the much more conclusive, though flawed, 1983 study.

Thinner *versus* Heavier: An Alternative View of the Evidence

The "definitive proof" that being thinner means living longer turns out to be dwarfed in comparison to a vast, globe-encircling body of evidence based on data that has been collected since the 1950s on hundreds of thousands of men and women of different ages, races, nationalities, and ethnicities. When this kind of more global, international approach is adopted, the vast majority of all the studies since the 1950s call that conclusion into question, either because they find weight to be irrelevant to health and mortality issues (except at the extremes of the Body Mass Index) or because, in some cases, BMI measurements that would currently be classified as overweight or obese appear to be the healthier ones, offering the best prospects for long life.

Consider, for example, the Seven Countries Study. Since the late 1950s and early 1960s researchers from around the world have been keeping track of the vital statistics of nearly thirteen thousand men in the United States, Finland, the Netherlands, Italy, Greece, Japan, and the former Yugoslavia, who were between the ages of forty and fifty-nine, and healthy, when they entered the study. Researchers took measurements of blood pressure, blood fats, height, weight, and other physiological data to assess their relationship to mortality data. Of the many reports that continue to be published from this ongoing study, none has shown that being thin offers any advantages in terms of life expectancy. On the contrary, a recent report on 7,985 Europeans in this study indicated that thin men (BMI less than 18.5) had a 25-year mortality rate—roughly twice that of men classified as either normal weight or overweight. This was true regardless of smoking status. Overweight (BMI between 25.0 and 29.9) had no impact on mortality. Although obesity did increase mortality risk relative to men in the normal or overweight BMI range, the death rate of fat men (BMI over 30) was lower than that of thin men.

The higher mortality among obese men in the Seven Countries Study is primarily due to coronary heart disease and stroke. With respect to cancer, however, higher BMIs are associated with *lower* mortality rates. "Relative body weight (body mass index) was an important negative risk factor, meaning that the risk of dying from cancer decreased with increasing relative weight."

Culturally diverse reports on causes of male mortality are certainly not limited to data issuing from the Seven Countries Study. There are many other long-range studies of young, middle-aged, and elderly men representing a variety of populations: civil service employees in Great Britain, Denmark, and Paris; German construction workers; middle-aged men in the British Regional Heart Study; Maoris in New Zealand; Pima Indians in Arizona; middle-aged men in Finland; middle-aged and older Japanese men; Italians participating in the Risk Factor and Life Expectancy project; San Francisco longshoremen; employees of the

Chicago Peoples Gas Company; residents of western Scotland; Californians in the Western Collaborative Group Study; state employees of New York in the Albany Study; older men in the Longitudinal Study of Aging; participants in the Epidemiological Follow-up Study of the first National Health and Nutrition Examination Survey (NHANES I); volunteers in the American Cancer Society's Cancer Prevention Study II; men living in California, Maryland, North Carolina, and Pennsylvania who were enrolled in the Cardiovascular Health Study; African Americans participating in the Charleston (South Carolina) Heart Study, the Evans County (Georgia) Heart Study, or the Kaiser Permanente Study in the San Francisco Bay area. All of these have produced results inconsistent with the notion that the thin live longest. Many have shown that weight has no independent impact on mortality, and a few have suggested that the heavy live longer.

Studies of women show similar results. For example, researchers at the University of Amsterdam conducted a twenty-five-year study of 1,464 middle-aged women living in the Netherlands that indicated that body weight is unrelated to premature death in both smokers and nonsmokers. Similarly a thirty-year evaluation of 741 white and 454 black women participating in the Charleston Heart Study showed no relationship between weight and mortality rates from heart disease. The same goes for the 2,731 black women tracked for fifteen years by researchers at the Kaiser Permanente Medical Care Program in Oakland, California— no relationship between weight and mortality rates, *for all causes of death.* From the standpoint of longevity, no study to date has shown thinner to be better than heavier for black women, not even at weights up to 59 BMI units, which constitutes extreme obesity. Conversely a twelve-year study of 17,159 Finnish women between the ages of twenty-five and seventy-nine showed an extraordinarily high mortality rate in very *thin* women—50 to 150 percent higher compared with women of average or slightly below average weight—regardless of whether or not they smoked. "It is noteworthy," the study remarked, "that the ill effects of thinness were evident not only among women who were extremely thin but also among those whose BMI was well within the range customarily considered as acceptable (20-25 BMI)."

The risks associated with thinness appear to be noted more frequently in older persons. In a study of 7,527 men and women age 70 and older, researchers at the University of Alabama found that the thinnest (BMI less than 19.4) had the highest mortality rates. Actually the heaviest men and women (BMI over 28.5) had the lowest death rates—even lower than those of normal weight. The researchers concluded that "obesity may be protective compared to thinness or normal weight in older community-dwelling Americans." A similar study of older community-dwelling women in Baltimore, Maryland showed the same thing, as did the results of the Cardiovascular Health Study, on 5,201 men and women of age 65 and over. Low body weight (less than 115 pounds for women and less than 142 pounds for men) was "strongly and independently predictive of mortality." The researchers also stressed that "overweight does not seem to be a risk factor for 5-year mortality in this age group." Many other studies from populations throughout the world reinforce these findings.

Critics, however, are quick to impugn studies that fail to show overweight to be unhealthy or that paint a bleak picture for the thin—although, as noted earlier, the vast majority of the studies conducted since the 1950s draw one or another of these conclusions. The critics have charged that these studies suffer from one or more of the following limitations: follow-up periods that are too short for the detrimental effects of overweight to be seen; failure to rule out the possibility that the high mortality of thin people seen in some of these studies may be attributable to smoking, which is usually more prevalent among the thin; failure to screen out thin people suffering from undetected diseases that, like cancer, may cause low weights or weight loss.

These criticisms do not hold up. As for the length of the follow-up, all of the studies I've mentioned have follow-up durations of between 10 and 30 years (with the exception of some of the studies on older persons, for whom a lengthy follow-up is not necessary to obtain statistically meaningful mortality data), with at least half a dozen lasting 20 years or more. These are comparable to the 1983 Framingham study, which made such a strong statement about the negative impact of weight, and was considerably longer than the life insurance studies, which, as noted, had an average follow-up period of 7.8 years for the 1959 study, and an even lower average of 6.6 for the 1979 study. Actually, of all the studies of weight and mortality that tracked a population for 20 years or longer, those that show thinner to be better are consistently outnumbered by those that show either that average, or heavier-than-average, weights are better or that weight has no impact one way or another on mortality.

The suggestion that thinness appeared as a risk factor for early mortality in so many of the studies only because it was often related to smoking can also be thoroughly rebutted. As mentioned above, in the study on Finnish women the high mortality rate among the thinnest women was unaffected by smoking. Similarly, a thirteen-year study of more than 20,000 Finnish men between the ages of twenty-five and seventy-nine found that thinness was consistently associated with mortality rates up to 4.7 times greater than men of average or above-average weight *among non-smokers.* Smoking also could not explain the fact that after sixteen years of tracking the 2,381 men between the ages of forty-five and seventy-five who were living in western Scotland, it was found that thin nonsmoking men had 40 percent higher death rates than men of average weight or above did.

Those studies in which thin men and women fare no better, and in some cases fare worse, than their average or heavier-than-average counterparts have been scrupulous about ruling out smoking as a possible cause for the mortality rates. This was made perfectly clear in a landmark report appearing in the *International Journal of Obesity* in 1996, on "The relationship between body weight and mortality: a quantitative analysis of combined information from existing studies." Researchers at the National Center for Health Statistics, and at Cornell University, scrutinized data from dozens of previously published studies, comprising a total of 356,747 men and 248,501 women, making it one of the most comprehensive analyses of the relationship between body weight and mortality published to date. Among nonsmoking men studied for up to 30 years, the relationship between BMI and mortality was U-shaped, with the lowest mortality rates observed between BMIs of 23 and 29. Thus, most of the BMI range that is considered overweight by current U.S. government weight guidelines (BMI 25 to 29.9) was not associated with higher risk. Low BMI, on the other hand, was.

Low BMI in this instance does not mean extremely thin. For example, mortality rates for men with BMIs between 19 and 21 (i.e., within the recommended range of U.S. government guidelines; for a 5' 10" man this would be approximately 130-145 pounds) were the same as for men with BMIs between 29 and 31 (i.e., extreme overweight or moderately obese; roughly 200-215 pounds for that same 5' 10" man). The researchers remarked, "This quantitative analysis of existing studies revealed increased mortality at moderately low BMI for white men comparable to that observed at extreme overweight, which does not appear to be due to smoking or existing disease. Attention to the health risks of underweight is needed, and body weight recommendations for optimum longevity need to be considered in light of these risks."

As for nonsmoking women, the researchers found no distinct minimum mortality point. The BMI range corresponding to the lowest death rates was quite large, stretching from about 18 all the way to 32, so a 5' 4" woman could weigh anywhere from 105 pounds to 185 pounds and have the same risk of premature death. Only beyond a BMI of 32 did the mortality rate begin to increase.

To refute the claim that some studies show higher mortality rates among the thin because they have failed to screen out those with undiagnosed diseases that cause weight loss, several recent long-term studies have reanalyzed their data to show that even when deaths that occurred in the first one to ten years of the study are omitted—deaths that might conceivably be due to illness that went undetected at the time the study began—the results are not materially altered. For example researchers at the NIH found that after eliminating deaths that occurred within the first seven years of a study of 1,034 elderly women who never smoked, their data showed that the thinnest women had a mortality rate 50 percent higher than women of average weight.

Data on 13,242 blacks and whites participating in the NHANES I Epidemiologic Follow-up Study, initiated in 1982, revealed that exclusion of persons with baseline illness and also persons who died within the first four years of follow-up did not change the results: a U-shaped relationship between BMI and mortality. The higher risk associated with thinness and obesity was noted for all groups, and was not influenced by smoking status. Among black men and women, the lowest mortality rates occurred at a BMI of about 27—in other words, overweight. Although minimum mortality in whites occurred at a BMI between 24 and 25, the researchers emphasized that in all groups studied there was a very broad BMI range of about 9 BMI units corresponding to only slightly elevated risk (20 percent or less). This translates to BMIs between approximately 22 and 31 for blacks and 20 and 29 for whites, and includes about 70 percent of the U.S. population. The authors of the study concluded that "the resulting empirical findings from each of four race/sex groups, which are representative of the US population, demonstrate a wide range of BMIs consistent with minimum mortality and do not suggest that the optimal BMI is at the lower end of the distribution for any subgroup."

The irony of the findings from this NIH-sponsored study is unmistakable, and calls into question the current U.S. government guidelines for body weight, *released by the NIH in 1998*, that recommend a BMI between 18.5 and 24.9 for optimum health and longevity. The NIH's *own data* demonstrate that at least part of that range—18.5 to about 20 for whites and 18.5 to about 22 for blacks—is worse in terms of longevity than being either overweight (for whites and blacks) or moderately obese (for blacks).

Potential Health Benefits
of Extra Pounds

There is a significant body of research that goes beyond telling us that weight does not really matter all that much, to suggest that carrying a few extra pounds, over and above the weights currently being recommended, may actually have health benefits, resulting in reduced risk of many diseases and disorders that affect quality as well as length of life. These diseases include lung cancer, the number-one cause of cancer deaths among men and women, premenopausal breast cancer, and osteoporosis. Excluding extremes, even weights currently defined as overweight or obese have been shown to have advantages.

By my count, there have been at least thirty-five to forty studies in the past thirty years or so that indicate a lower incidence of cancer, and of mortality from cancer, at higher body weights. Lung cancer is one of the diseases where the benefits are particularly noticeable. Besides the Seven Countries Study, mentioned above, there is also a most impressive set of results from a National Cancer Institute-sponsored study of 3,607 lung cancer patients, ranging in age from twenty to eighty, who were compared with a control group of 9,681. The most dramatic findings concerned the women subjects: Among those who had never smoked, women with a BMI between 22 and 24.9 had a 140 percent higher risk of developing lung cancer than women with a BMI of 28 or more. In other words, it was better to be clinically overweight or obese than within recommended guidelines. Thin women (BMI less than 22) had the greatest risk—190 percent higher than women with a BMI of 28 or more did.

A number of other studies show similar results, all of them well-designed studies that have looked at smokers and nonsmokers separately and have ruled out deaths in the early years of the follow-up period, thus ensuring that deaths due to illnesses undiagnosed at the time the study began (including those illnesses associated with thinness) would be screened out. Drs. Geoffrey Kabat and Ernst Wynder, co-authors of the National Cancer Institute-sponsored study, assessed all the literature on the subject and reported that "The overall consistency in the inverse association of body mass with lung cancer in reported studies is impressive. *It is noteworthy that no study shows a significant contrary trend.*" (Italics mine.)

Breast cancer in premenopausal women is another of the diseases for which extra weight seems to be an advantage. In a combined analysis of seven studies—four from the United States, including the Nurses' Health Study, and one each from Canada, Sweden, and the Netherlands—involving 337,819 women, researchers found that premenopausal breast cancer rates decreased as BMI increased. Women with BMI of 31 or greater had a 46 percent lower risk of developing breast cancer than women with a BMI of 21 or less had. Similar results have been reported in several other large-scale studies, including one from Norway which numbered 570,000 women. In addition to the benefit of a high BMI, weight gain from young adulthood to middle age appears to be associated with reduced risk of premenopausal breast cancer. The Nurses' Health Study, for example, found that premenopausal women who had gained more than forty-four pounds since the age of eighteen had a 40 percent lower risk of developing breast cancer than women who had gained or lost less than about seven pounds. These results seem to have been forgotten in the rush to judgment that occurred with the release of the Nurses' Health Study data on cardiovascular disease.

It is only fair to mention that for postmenopausal women, most, but certainly not all, studies show a BMI association with breast cancer that is opposite to that observed for premenopausal women. However, the increased risk associated with high BMI in postmenopausal women is less (typically no more than 20-30 percent) than the elevated risk associated with thinness among premenopausal women (generally 40-50 percent). Consequently, the lifetime risk of breast cancer—most of which occurs after menopause—may not be affected appreciably by BMI. In a 2000 report on the "Cumulative risk of breast cancer to age 70 years according to risk factor analysis," Nurses' Health Study researchers found little difference in cumulative lifetime incidence of breast cancer when comparing average women (who gained 19 pounds from ages 18 to 50) with women who remained relatively weight stable during their adult lives, and also with women who were either consistently lean or consistently obese during their adult lives. Appreciably higher cumulative lifetime breast cancer risk was only observed in women who experienced significant adult weight gain (60 pounds or more).

The association between high BMI and postmenopausal breast cancer risk is confounded by a number of factors, including exercise and hormone replacement therapy. Postmenopausal hormone replacement therapy usually is associated with increased breast cancer risk, as was generally the case in the Nurses' Health Study. Interestingly, in this study high BMI was linked to increased breast cancer risk only in postmenopausal women who were *not using* hormone replacement therapy. Overweight and obese postmenopausal women who *did receive* hormone replacement therapy actually had a *lower* cumulative breast cancer risk, similar to that of premenopausal women. Further research is necessary to determine why hormone replacement therapy might "protect" against breast cancer only in postmenopausal women with high BMIs.

Exercise also has been shown to reduce the risk of postmenopausal breast cancer. One recent report from the NHANES I Epidemiological Follow-up Study found that a consistently high level of recreational activity was associated with a 67 percent reduction in breast cancer risk. This suggests that the modestly increased postmenopausal breast cancer risk associated with high BMI might be offset by a physically active lifestyle.

How to account for the association between high BMI and lower risk of certain cancers is as yet unclear. There are, however, several distinct possibilities. Data from the 1971-1974 National Health and Nutrition Examination Survey in the United States (NHANES I), as well as from the Central American Nutrition Survey, suggest that the cancer rates may have something to do with the fact that men and women who weigh more consume more of the anticarcinogen beta carotene. In a study of 25,994 Finnish men, researchers found that consumption of vegetables and antioxidants was greatest—and lung cancer rates lowest—among men with the highest BMIs. As for survival rates, the better survival statistics for certain cancers in heavy people may be related to the fact that they have more abundant stores of energy (body fat) to call upon, particularly during such demanding treatments as chemotherapy.

Another major disease for which being heavy appears as a distinct advantage, in terms of both incidence and seriousness, is osteoporosis, a bone-wasting disease that afflicts an estimated 20 to 25 million Americans, mainly women over the age of forty-five. But it's not confined to that age group, as suggested by hip fracture rates that start to rise dramatically in the forty- to forty-four-year-olds—22 per 100,000, compared with 3 per 100,000 in the thirty-five- to thirty-nine-year-olds. Characterized by deterioration of bone mineral density, osteoporosis greatly increases the risk of bone fractures, some 1.5 million of which, mostly of the vertebra and hip, are directly attributed to osteoporosis each year. Such fractures can be extremely serious, with the mortality rate from hip fracture complications, for example, going as high as 50 percent among those sixty-five and over. Fewer than half of those who suffer hip fractures ever fully recover. In fact, hip fracture is a major cause of disability among North American women, with thin women being more than twice as vulnerable to the problem as heavy women. In the United Kingdom, the Osteoporosis Society reports that more women die from hip fractures due to osteoporosis than from cancers of the cervix, uterus, and breast *combined*.

The heavier you are, the less likely you are to suffer from the demineralization of the bone that is involved in osteoporosis. Why this is so is still a matter of speculation, but hormonal, mechanical, and nutritional factors may all play a part. Heavy women tend to have higher estrogen levels in their blood, which protects against bone loss, and there may continue to be some estrogen production in fat tissue even after menopause. Also, heavy women typically consume more food than thin women do, which may provide a greater nutrient supply for optimal bone health. From a mechanical standpoint, "The strong effect of weight on bone mineral density is due to load on weight-bearing bones in both sexes." This finding is from yet another of the unpublicized reports from the Framingham study that suggests that relatively high body weights, as well as weight gain over the years, have definite advantages. A number of other studies, including two at the Mayo Clinic, one at Tufts, and one in France, to mention just a few, show similar results for osteoporosis. As the French researchers concluded, "Even moderate obesity can play a protective role on postmenopausal bone loss."

None of this should be taken as a recommendation to attempt to gain weight in order to reduce the risks associated with this bone-wasting disease, but it does undermine certain basic assumptions about the evils of weight. It also challenges the indiscriminate recommendation to lose weight for better health, because dieting has been shown to increase the likelihood of losing bone mass. It is sobering to realize that the thinness we worship and the diets we go on to try to achieve it may be increasing the risk of incurring a debilitating, and potentially life-threatening, disease.

Other diseases for which being heavy appears to be an advantage, either in terms of developing them or surviving them, include infectious diseases such as tuberculosis, and respiratory diseases such as emphysema, chronic obstructive lung disease, and bronchitis. Heavy men and women with hypertension have better survival rates than their thinner counterparts, perhaps because of different cardiovascular dynamics (as was explained in Chapter 3). Among type 2 diabetics, those with a BMI in the "overweight" range have considerably lower death rates than those with an average, or below average, BMI.

The list of possible advantages goes on. The attentive reader, though, will want to know whether the apparent health benefits of being heavy are directly attributed to the weight and/or the body fat itself or to other factors, with which weight may have a merely incidental association. After all, even the explanations proffered for most of the cancer and osteoporosis benefits are still speculative and subject to alternate interpretations.

Just as I have criticized studies that identify low body weight as a critical or key variable for reduced risk of certain diseases and disorders, I must caution that heavier body weights may not be the key factor to account for the lower incidence or mortality rates for the conditions mentioned above, however close the association may be. Few, if any, studies to date have been carefully enough designed to focus on weight while simultaneously excluding other likely influences on health and well-being. It may be that in those studies indicating a possible causal relationship between body weight and various diseases—whether it's low weight or high weight that is seen as the problem—the weight itself is not the important factor, but some other as yet unnoted and unmeasured variable, which also happens to affect body weight.

My point is that definitive proof of any given hypothesis about the weight-health correlation is almost impossible at the present time. The prevailing assumptions are based largely on the extremely flawed studies by the life insurance industry, studies that are directly contradicted by a vast amount of evidence from better designed, more rigorously controlled, and longer-range studies. But change comes very slowly to the medical and scientific establishment. It took nearly half a century for the actuarial data to be accepted, and now that they have been accepted, who knows how much longer they will remain the basis of our beliefs? At the moment, "thinner is healthier" is the popular gospel; anything else is heresy.

Hence the continuing faith we put in the ubiquitous height-weight tables. However, a careful look at them will reveal a multitude of problems. It's not just the actuarial data on which they are based that are flawed; the tables have their own flaws, based on unwarranted assumptions and interpretations that are specific to them.

CHAPTER 5

"Ideal" Height-Weight Tables:
Measuring the Immeasurable

The fact is that the tables of 'ideal' or 'desirable' weight are arm-chair concoctions starting with questionable assumptions and ending with three sets of standards for 'body frames' which were never measured or even properly defined. Unfortunately, those tables have been reprinted by the thousands and are widely accepted as the gospel truth.

—Ancel Keys, Professor Emeritus, University of Minnesota,
Nutrition Reviews, 1980

In Greek mythology it was the custom of an outlaw named Procrustes to offer shelter to travelers who happened by his house in Attica, near the road to Athens. Procrustes had but one request of his guests— that they sleep in his bed. The problem was that the travelers came in many sizes, and Procrustes' bed in only one—and Procrustes insisted on a perfect fit. This posed no problem for those lucky enough to be the right size, but created a rather inhospitable ordeal for those who were not: Short guests were stretched out on a rack until they were long enough to fit; tall guests had their legs sawed off to the appropriate length.

Procrustes would have loved the height-weight tables. Like his bed, they are arbitrary, refusing to take into account the considerable and natural variations in human body size and shape. Also like his bed, they have created unnecessary agony for those who do not "fit." The "ideal" or "desirable" weights they prescribe are our modern form of mythology. When I say that they are an attempt to measure the immeasurable, I am not referring to the height and weight variables themselves, which are easily measurable. Instead, I am referring to the idea that the "ideal" can be measured, that it can be presented in terms of a fixed number of pounds (or range of pounds) that shows up on a height-weight table, and that that number should be presented as having a universal application.

Weight Tables: Arbitrary, Random, and Meaningless

It *is* likely that for each person there is a particular weight, or range of weights, that can be considered healthy, but that weight is not necessarily going to appear on any height-weight tables currently in existence, or likely to be. Tables of "ideal" or "desirable" weights make about as much sense as tables of ideal or desirable heights. Actually, in view of how the height-weight tables were created, they make no sense at all.

As discussed in Chapter 2, Met Life's passionate antiobesity advocate, Louis Dublin, was the principal creator of the 1942-43 tables, which have been a major influence on our thinking about weight ever since. Those tables were the first to suggest that weight gain after one's twenties was unhealthy, a conclusion Dublin apparently arrived at based on the low mortality rates of people in their twenties, which he believed to be connected to their relatively low body weights. But that's only the beginning of the problems with the tables he created.

Dublin noticed that for any given height there was a considerable range of weights that appeared to be associated with low mortality. In most instances apparently healthy weights could span a range as broad as thirty to forty pounds. Since this did not conform well with the concept of a specific weight that was "ideal" or "desirable," Dublin resolved his dilemma by reasoning that the wide range of weights must be explained by differences in skeletal frame sizes. With that notion in mind, he split the weight range into thirds, connecting small frames with poundages at the light end of the weight range, medium frames with medium weights, and large frames with the heavier weights. Though this seems logical, it has never been established in any scientific way, nor has frame size in the insured ever been measured in any scientific way.

Nor is this by any means the end of the flaws in the tables. Another piece of apparent "logic" that characterizes the height-weight tables is the perfectly linear manner in which the tables progress through height and frame sizes, with regular and proportional increases in recommended weight cropping up at each increase in the other dimensions. While this does indeed seem logical, it does not reflect the findings of the actuarial data on which Met Life's tables are supposedly based, leaving aside the question that was explored in the last chapter, of whether the studies that generated those data are seriously flawed.

To illustrate, consider a couple of examples from the most recent edition of the Met Life tables, dating from 1983, and based on the 1979 Build Study. The Met Life tables of 1983 show only one age group: 25-59. The Build Study tables have six age groups, starting with 15-19-year-olds, then progressing in increments of ten years: 20-29, 30-39 and so forth to age 69; and of several inches: 4'11" to 5'2", 5'3"-5'6", and so forth. For a fifty-five-year-old woman who is 5'4" tall, and of small or medium frame, the Met Life tables indicate that the recommended weight is between 114 pounds and 138 pounds. However, according to data published in the actual Build Study, on a table entitled "Mortality Experience for Women by Age Group... According to Height and Weight," part of that recommended weight range, 114-124, would put that woman in a higher-than-standard mortality group. Conversely the weight at which she would have the lowest of all mortality rates, would be—and this is hard to believe but written in black and white—185-194. Similarly, a woman in her forties, 5'2", should weigh not less than 108 nor more than 143 pounds, depending on frame size, according to the Met Life tables. But the Build Study reveals that her lowest mortality rate would occur between 155 and 164. For both the 5'2" and 5'4" heights, the Build Study shows lowest mortality rates at weights considered clinically overweight or obese. Though I have chosen two of the more dramatic sets of discrepancies between Met Life and Build Study tables, there are numerous discrepancies for both men and women, in virtually all height and age groups.

The discrepancies tend to get more extreme with age, which is why I used for my examples women in their forties and fifties. The weight associated with lowest mortality for a forty-five-year-old is not necessarily the same as that for a twenty-five-year-old. It is, in fact, higher. According to the 1979 Build Study, from about middle age on, the weights that correspond to the lowest death rates are frequently well in excess of Met Life's recommended range, sometimes extending into weights considered very overweight. This was one of the points made by Dr. Reubin Andres, clinical director of the National Institute on Aging, when he explained the results of his own statistical analysis of the Build Study. The "age-independent" tables generated by Met Life had erred, he said, "apparently in an effort to simplify the weight recommendations, by not entering age as a variable."

There is no denying that the death rates of older and typically heavier men and women are higher than the death rates of their younger and typically lighter counterparts, but the rates are higher primarily because of *age*, not the pounds that frequently accompany the aging process. All we learn from the life insurance data is that as you get older, you are more likely to die—not exactly an earth-shattering revelation. It's safe to say that age is the single best predictor of mortality.

Why the 1983 Met Life tables are such an inaccurate reflection of the 1979 Build Study data is hard to say. But one guess is that it has to do with the fact that it's impossible to construct a coherent table on the basis of those data. If you look at the Build Study table for women in their forties who stand 5'7" to 5'10", for example, there is a column expressing the ratio (percentage) of actual to expected mortality, with 100 standing for the expected rate, anything under 100 being less than expected, and over 100 being more. At weights of 115-124 the ratio is 68—considerably lower than expected. It is also the lowest on the chart for that height, suggesting that these weights are very good weights indeed for those women; at 125-134 the rate goes up to 108—bad; at 135-144 it goes down to 87—good, though not as great as 115-124. Looking at these charts and how those mortality ratios jump around without any apparent regard for orderly weight progressions, which is what we like to see on our charts, one is struck by how utterly random the associations between weight and mortality seem to be. At first glance it may seem that at the bottom of the charts, where the heaviest weights appear, the mortality rates do seem to go consistently up, suggesting that those weights are indeed a mortality risk. However, a closer look reveals such anomalies as the 5'3"-5'6", 185-194-pound woman in her fifties whose mortality ratio is 77—very low indeed. Yet her 195-204-pound sister is at the predictably high mortality ratio of 134. No wonder Met Life may have felt the need to "simplify weight recommendations."

What does it all mean? Probably nothing. A few minutes of looking at the Build Study tables might be enough to convince one of the meaninglessness of weight as a predictor of mortality. But what is the harm in the various height-weight tables, one might ask, since they do serve as a much-needed reminder to many of us that we are eating too much of the wrong foods and exercising too little? To begin with, there is the unquestionable fact that the tables unjustly penalize and cause unnecessary anguish in men and women who have natural body weights outside the recommended range. Many of them will engage in all kinds of extreme and unhealthy dieting behavior that will never get them to the weight they want to be, much less allow them to maintain it, and may end by making them heavier. Then there are the numerous smokers (mostly women) who refuse to give up the habit because of their fear of possible weight gain—a fate apparently worse than death in many people's minds. Many young girls start smoking in an effort to control their weight.

Furthermore, reliance on the tables may cause people who do fall within the weight guidelines to continue engaging in an unhealthy lifestyle, out of a false sense of security. I have talked with many men and women who insist, "I don't need to exercise because I don't have a weight problem" or who proclaim, "I can eat anything I want because I never gain weight." Yet millions of men and women who suffer from diseases resulting in premature death—diseases that a healthier lifestyle might help to prevent—have body weights perfectly in line with height-weight table recommendations.

Individualized Ideal Body Weights and Set Points

None of this is meant to suggest that there is no such thing as an ideal weight. As explained before, for each person there is such a weight, or weight range, but the height-weight tables are not the place to find it. How, then, will you know if you're there? The absolutely honest answer to this question is that you may never know for certain. The best guesstimate, though, is that you are probably at your ideal weight when you are not trying to do anything to control your weight, but *are* eating a relatively low-fat, fiber-rich diet abundant in fruits, vegetables, and whole grains, and being physically active.

Trying to say anything beyond that about an ideal weight is impossible, because the ideal for each person is unique to him or her, thanks to the unique genetic makeup of each person's body. One critical aspect of that uniqueness is the set point, which is the body weight (or perhaps body fat percentage) that each person's body tends to maintain over long periods of time, regardless of whether that weight is a good weight or a bad weight. This probably explains why so many people maintain stable weights without even trying, and why millions of others keep returning to more or less the same weight despite perpetual efforts to diet. Though we don't fully understand what is being "set" by the set point, we do know that it exists, and that it operates with a good deal of precision. If it did not, the consequences would be rather striking.

Consider, for example, a typical woman who consumes an average of 2,000 calories per day. Over a period of one year this would be nearly three-quarters of a million calories. We assume that for this woman's weight not to change, the number of calories burned needs to match the number of calories consumed. But it is most unlikely that there would be such a neat match between input and output. Let us say, then, that the difference between the two was 1 percent more calories consumed than burned—a plausible scenario given the increasingly sedentary lifestyle of most people as they age. This would add up to 7,300 calories, or the equivalent of about 2 pounds of body fat per year. If this imbalance continued unchecked in the weight gain direction, which is, after all, the direction most of us go in, it would result in a gain of about 20 pounds per decade, or more than 100 pounds during the course of her adult lifetime. Yet it would be rare indeed for a 125-pound twenty-year-old to end up at 225 pounds by the time she's a senior citizen.

There is clearly some mechanism within each of us that functions fairly well to keep body weight reasonably constant over long periods of time. How that works, and why it varies so much from person to person, such that one woman will have her weight "set" at 120, another at 150, and another at 175, can best be understood by looking at the tremendous variations that occur in muscle and fat content.

In general we can say that muscle and fat combined make up well over one-half of each person's body weight, with skin, bones, blood, and organs making up most of the rest; and that men's bodies typically have a higher ratio of muscle to fat than women's do. Individual variations in the amount of muscle and fat tissue, and consequently in the amount of body weight, are determined by both number and size of muscle and fat cells. Someone with a great number of large-sized muscle and/or fat cells will weigh more than someone with fewer, smaller cells. As to the question of why there are such variations from one person to the next, the answer lies, in large part, in our genes.

The number of muscle cells each one of us has is determined before birth, remains basically the same throughout life (with some decrease in our senior years), and for the most part is beyond our control. What does change, and what is partly within our control, is the size of those cells. There is a natural, steady increase in size that occurs as part of our normal growth from infancy to childhood and adolescence. That growth pattern culminates in the achievement of adult-sized cells, usually sometime in our late teens. Thereafter the size of the cells is affected most by use. If we become couch potatoes and don't use our muscles, the cells tend to shrink from atrophy; if we become bodybuilders and overload them by intense physical activity, they will grow larger from hypertrophy. If we engage in moderate amounts of occasional physical activity, such as recreational sports and aerobic exercise, the muscle cells remain basically the same size.

Fat cells have a more complicated destiny, dependent on a more intricate interplay of lifestyle and genetics, and they also have more impact on body weight, especially on the weight gain that most Americans typically experience as they age. Each of us is born with a given number of fat cells, which ranges somewhere between about 5 and 10 billion. These baby-sized fat cells grow considerably in size during the first year of life, with most of their growth being achieved by the end of that year, at which time they can be said to have reached the size of fat cells found in adults. Though the size of the cells will still be subject to change after that, depending on various lifestyle factors, the biggest change will be in number, not in size, for the number of cells keeps increasing dramatically throughout childhood and adolescence. Thus, by the time a boy or girl reaches the age of about twenty, the number of fat cells can range from around 20 billion in a lean person to 100 billion or more in a very fat person. Most people fall somewhere in between.

The reason for the wide variation in the number of fat cells produced during the growing period is not entirely understood, but appears to be largely a matter of genes. The genetic component of our fat makeup is, so far as we know, unalterable. If one person is genetically programmed to have twice the number of fat cells that someone else does, then it can only be expected that that first person will have a set point for body fat, and body weight, that is much higher than the second person's. For millions this higher set point has resulted in weights that are above height-weight table recommendations. They are not inherently less healthy than other people, just *inherently heavier*.

Are we, then, prisoners of our genes, unalterably destined to be thin or fat depending on genetic programming? To a certain extent this would seem to be the case, though there is some compelling evidence from experiments done on laboratory animals to suggest that the proliferation of fat cells during our growth years can be influenced by exercise and nutrition. Though no such direct evidence exists for human beings, since no experiments have been done, it nonetheless makes sense to encourage children to be as physically active as possible and to discourage them from eating junk foods loaded with fat and sugar. Whether this will alter their ultimate fat-quotient destiny can only be surmised, but they will almost certainly be healthier as a result. The evidence we do have— research done at Harvard, for example —shows that among children there is a strong relation between TV watching and obesity.

The Fattening of America: Set-Point Alteration and Weight Change

One thing we know for certain about fat cells: Once we've got them, they're ours to keep. The number of fat cells can always continue to go up, but never down. Why this is so—why we continue to experience increases in fat-cell number during adulthood, often quite significant increases—is only a matter of speculation at this point, but both genes and lifestyle are believed to play a part. About the genetic component of the set point there is nothing to be done, obviously. As far as we know, however, the body's set point does not *necessarily* shift to a higher weight as we age, thereby programming the body to get fatter. It's the typical late-twentieth-century American way of life that is probably the major culprit in the tendency of most men and women to put on twenty or more pounds during their adult years—pounds that are almost always the result of both adding new fat cells and packing more fat into each individual cell. Since lifestyle can be changed, fat stores can also be changed, *within limits.*

Given that we can grow more fat cells, but not get rid of them, the only way to lose fat is by reducing the amount of fat in our existing cells. Such reductions can occur, and so can the reverse. Whether the amount of fat in each fat cell increases, decreases, or remains the same is greatly affected by two things: exercise and the type—not necessarily the amount—of food we eat. The body's natural tendency is to store fat when it's fed fat, because it is not a particularly good fat burner. By contrast, it is an excellent burner of carbohydrates. A person who eats a high-fat diet and changes the ratio of carbohydrates to fat, switching to a low-fat, high-complex-carbohydrate regimen, will reduce the amount of fat in each fat cell, even if the total number of calories consumed remains the same or is actually increased modestly, and will reduce it still more with the fat-burning effects of exercise. Conversely, physical inactivity and a diet high in fats and sugars will increase the amount of fat in each cell.

As explained above, these changes do not indicate a defect in the set point, for the set point can itself change—good news for those who feel themselves to be at a weight that is not natural to them, a weight that could be improved by engaging in a healthier way of life. Such an approach certainly worked for Mark, a former graduate student of mine in the Exercise Physiology Program at the University of Virginia.

In his late teens, Mark had weighed close to 350 pounds—a very hefty weight indeed, even for a six-foot-tall man. He had always been heavy and over the course of several years had tried numerous diets at the recommendations of several different doctors and dietitians. Nothing worked. The weight of 350 pounds—the highest ever for him—was all he had to show for his dieting experiences. He was miserable about his weight, which everyone around him found unattractive, and the physical effort of carrying so many pounds made him feel slow, tired, clumsy, and uncomfortable. Discouraged by his multiple dieting "failures," he decided to try something new. Instead of cutting calories he would focus on cutting the amount of fat in his diet. He reduced his fat consumption to about 10 percent of the total calories he ate each day—a far cry from the typical American menu. Over a period of about one year, he lost 160 pounds, reaching a weight of 190. Though he was now close—the closest he had ever been—to falling within the guidelines of the height-weight tables, he felt miserable and weak at this weight.

At this point he decided that in order to regain strength and vitality, he would relax his restrictions on dietary fat, upping his fat allowance to about 20 percent of total calories, and he would begin exercising more—mainly lifting weights. He gained some weight back, finally settling at about 225 pounds, a weight he has maintained for the past five years. He feels great, exercises daily, and eats plenty of low-fat foods. Most importantly, Mark never goes hungry and eats as often as he likes—sometimes six or seven times a day.

Mark's case is extraordinary only in terms of the *amount* of weight he lost. The *manner* in which he lost it, and eventually regained some to arrive at his current, comfortable weight of 225 pounds, felt natural and even easy. Anyone who feels overly heavy could follow the recommendation to "be active and eat less fat" and find his or her way to a healthier weight. Low-fat eating and higher levels of physical activity force fat cells to give up some of their fat, which results in loss of weight.

But there's a catch. The number of fat cells won't diminish, and the size of a fat cell can only get so low, and that's it. While some people may have lower set points for the amount of fat in each cell, for each of us there is some limit, which no amount of lifestyle improvement is going to be able to change. Thus, setting specific weight-loss goals becomes an exercise in futility. Weight loss for the sake of arriving at some arbitrary, predetermined weight is pointless, because it places value on something that is worthless as a measure of health. Let's look again at Mark's experience.

What is Mark's "ideal" weight? Who knows. From a health perspective it's impossible to tell. He has no overt health problems now, at 225 pounds, nor did he have any at 350 or at 190. But he didn't feel comfortable at either the 350 or the 190 weights, and he does feel good at 225, even though he is still clinically obese, at a BMI of over 30. Since this is the weight that Mark's body seems to have selected after he began living healthfully, and this is a weight at which he feels energetic and strong, it is probably safe to say that it is compatible with his set point and the other two weights weren't. Perhaps at 190 pounds his naturally generous endowment of muscle and fat tissue had shrunk to levels that were, *for him*, abnormally low and unhealthy, which was why he felt too tired to enjoy life and could hardly muster enough energy to engage in any exercise. At 350 he was probably well above his set point, because of a complex interplay of factors, including stress-related eating, and the yo-yo dieting he did to counteract the results.

Having followed my advice to ignore the height-weight tables, Mark was surprised and a bit insulted when I informed him that, at 225 he is considered obese by current medical and scientific guidelines. This point brings us to the crux of the problem. Such guidelines, and the health practitioners and doctors who issue them, do not take into account individual variations in set point. They put an overweight label on millions of fat people whose fat cells are numerous but happen to be at a "healthy" size, and they give a false sense of security to millions of thin and average-weight people with relatively few fat cells, all of which may be bursting at the seams, thanks to a daily regimen of too much junk food and too little exercise. No wonder there are so many studies that find little or no relationship between body weight and health.

Body Fat Has Gotten a Bad Rap

Perhaps it's becoming clear that obesity is not a major killer, thinner is not necessarily healthier or longer lived, and the height-weight tables don't measure anything meaningful. An even more persistent part of our health mythology is the belief that body fat is intrinsically bad. Nearly seventy years ago, Dr. Woods Hutchinson, former president of the American Medical Association, remarked that he was baffled by what he felt at the time was an "onslaught upon one of the most peaceful, useful, and law-abiding of our tissues."

Little has changed since then, though we now believe with equal fervency that lean tissue, specifically muscle tissue, is good. Ask any health professional about weight loss and he or she will tell you that the goal is to lose body fat and minimize the loss of lean body tissue (defined as all other tissue on the body except fat). Even those of us who no longer look to the scale for confirmation of our health status may only have traded in that belief for a reliance on one of the many high-tech measures of body fat.

These beliefs notwithstanding, body fat is not intrinsically unhealthy tissue, and having a lot of it is not a death sentence. Depending on certain variables that will be explained in the next chapter, it may be a harbinger of a long and healthy life because all body fat is not alike. Some fat has been identified as providing protection from degenerative diseases, including, most notably, atherosclerosis. Yet there is also some body fat that has been shown to be undeniably hazardous. We need to understand the difference between *good* body fat and *bad* body fat, how this difference may affect health, and what we can do about it.

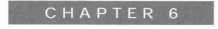

CHAPTER 6

Good Body Fat, *Bad* Body Fat

It is suggested that, not only does advice on the subject of obesity need reappraisal, but that research into possible associated benefits of moderate obesity would be worthwhile.

—Reubin Andres, M.D., Clinical Director, National Institute on Aging, *International Journal of Obesity*, 1980

Benefits of moderate obesity?! With attitudes about body fat being what they are, it is fair to say that the very notion sounds preposterous. But time has proven the wisdom of Dr. Andres' recommendation, and the research efforts are beginning to bear fruit. Not that one would know it from a review of the popular literature on the subject, however. A trip to the library to look up information on the possible advantages of moderate obesity will almost certainly be in vain. We have been thoroughly conditioned to believe that when it comes to weight in general and body fat in particular, less is always better. That message also comes through in the media.

The fallacy of that perception has been exposed in the previous chapters. There is more to the story, however, because with respect to body fat, both "less" and "more" can be better. It all depends on where it is. In this regard body fat is like real estate, with respect to which there are only three things that are said to matter: location, location, and location. It's not how much body fat you have, but where you have it that is important.

Take Lucy, for example, a thirty-year-old woman I encountered in the cardiovascular health and fitness program at the University of Virginia. She is a very physically active woman who carries about 95 pounds of body fat on her 5'5" frame. At an overall weight of 206 pounds, her body is roughly 46 percent fat, which is about twice as much fat— 95 pounds—as the average adult woman in the United States has. But does twice as much fat mean twice the health risks? Not if you look at any of the indices of health that we've been discussing in previous chapters, including total cholesterol (which in Lucy's case is a considerably below-average 150 mg/dl), HDL cholesterol and LDL cholesterol levels, triglyceride level, blood glucose level, and blood pressure, which all happen to be just fine, and have been for years. Lucy has no overt health problems at all, despite carrying around all that "excess" fat.

How a woman could carry almost half of her total weight in the form of fat—and a very substantial amount of weight it is—and not be at death's door would seem to be a mystery. However, it so happens that Lucy, like most women, carries a lot of her body fat on her hips and thighs, unlike most men, who usually carry more of their fat around their waist. Therein may lie a key to Lucy's good health and to the fact that women, despite having proportionately more body fat than men, live longer lives. Total *amounts*, or percentages, of body fat seem by most criteria of health to be relatively meaningless. *Location* of body fat, by contrast, can be very informative.

Keep this in mind the next time you go to a health club or fitness center that offers body fat testing to its clients. No matter how it is done—underwater weighing, skin fold, bioelectrical impedance, ultrasound—or how accurate the result is claimed to be, don't bother with it, and certainly don't pay for it. As these tests are currently performed, they may tell you how *much* fat you have, but not where it is located. From a health perspective this is worthless information. It doesn't tell you what you really want to know: whether your body fat location makes you an "apple" or a "pear." (*That* you can determine with the help of a tape measure and a couple of diagrams that are provided later in this chapter.)

Pears and Apples

Lucy is a "pear." She has what Professor Jean Vague of the University of Marseilles first described back in the 1940s as a typically gynoid, or female, distribution of body fat, with most of her visible fat on her thighs and hips. The typically android, or male, distribution is characterized by relatively more fat around the belly than below the waist—an apple shape. While these are the typical shapes for men and women, there are always exceptions, with many women being apple-shaped, and many men pear-shaped.

In both his clinical experience with patients and his scientific research studies, Dr. Vague noticed that *where* a person stored body fat revealed a lot about his or her physical well-being. For example, pear-shaped women seemed to have remarkably fewer health complications—a lower incidence of heart disease, diabetes, and gout, to name a few—than women whose body shapes more closely resembled an apple. Unfortunately it took more than three decades for Dr. Vague's seminal observations to make an impact on the medical and scientific communities of the United States—decades during which our antiobesity mania was skyrocketing.

Finally, in the 1980s, Dr. Vague's work began to attract some notice here, sparking interest among a number of scientists. A research team at the Medical College of Wisconsin, in Milwaukee, confirmed the French researcher's findings: Compared with women with a predominantly lower-body accumulation of fat, women with mostly upper-body fat had much higher risks for diabetes and heart disease, in the form of abnormal glucose metabolism and elevated body fat levels. Since these findings first appeared, research on the health impact of body fat location has accelerated dramatically, giving rise to the apple/pear distinction, which is now known to the public at large, not just to a few researchers in the field.

When first introduced to a lay audience, the idea that an apple-shaped body indicated a greatly increased risk for such major diseases as atherosclerosis and diabetes found a ready acceptance, because it still bore a "fat is bad" message that the public felt comfortable with. That a pear-shaped distribution of fat might mean *good* things for one's metabolic and cardiovascular health was not so readily accepted, however. Instead the message to pears was that their body fat was *relatively* benign, that it did not carry with it *as much* risk. Nevertheless, *some* risk was implied. After all, given the mainstream view of obesity, it seemed implausible that lots of fat, no matter where it was located, could actually do a person some good.

Notwithstanding this prejudice, in the past 15 years or so researchers have accumulated impressive evidence to the effect that a bountiful store of fat on hips and thighs is associated with a lower risk of heart disease and type 2 diabetes in both men and women. It has been shown that plentiful hip and thigh fat can even overcome the usual association between the apple shape and bad blood-fat profiles. Consider the following studies:

- In 1991 researchers at Stanford University found that among 133 men and 130 women between the ages of twenty-five and forty-nine, the bigger the thighs, the lower their heart disease risks. A relatively large thigh circumference, especially in women, was associated with healthfully low levels of blood triglycerides and LDL cholesterol (the bad kind, which promotes heart disease), and high levels of HDL cholesterol (the good kind, which protects against heart disease). Men and women with small thigh circumferences had just the opposite blood-fat profile. To make sure that it was thigh *fat*, and not muscle or bone, that was mainly responsible for the size of the thighs, the researchers then used a high-tech procedure called dual-photon absorptiometry to accurately determine the amount of fat in the thighs of eighty-one of the men and sixty-six of the women, and redid their statistical analysis focusing on thigh *fat* rather than thigh circumference. The results were the same: *The fatter the better.*

- In 1992 researchers at Laval University in Quebec used CAT scans (computerized axial tomography) to show that, among fifty-eight young men with a predominantly apple shape, generous amounts of thigh fat seemed to counteract the high-risk blood-fat profile that was typical of that body configuration. The men with the fattest thighs had the lowest levels of blood triglycerides, for example, and the highest levels of HDL cholesterol. Once again, *the fatter the thighs, the better the blood-fat profiles.*

- In the 1980s researchers at the Medical College of Wisconsin published two reports stemming from a large-scale study of more than seventy-six thousand U.S. and Canadian women enrolled in local chapters of TOPS (Take Off Pounds Sensibly). Each woman filled out a comprehensive health questionnaire and also provided the researchers with information regarding height, weight, and various girth measurements, including the hips. If they looked just at height-weight measurements, the researchers found the usual: at any given height, the heavier women tended to have a higher prevalence of diabetes and high blood pressure, as well as gallbladder disease. When other measurements were factored in, the connection between weight and health became more complicated. It was noted, for example, that "mildly obese" women who were pear-shaped had only half the prevalence of diabetes as "nonobese" women with slender hips. To determine whether there was a separate and independent association between hip circumference and diabetes, high blood pressure, and gallbladder disease, the researchers further analyzed their data by doing a statistical analysis that eliminated other body dimensions (comparative weight and waist size) as a possible factor. In every instance the results were the same: Pears fared better. *The larger the hips, the lower the risk.*

- A 1998 report from the Nurses' Health Study affirmed the health benefit of a pear shape, this time for coronary heart disease. Among 44,702 middle-aged women studied for eight years, the combination of large hips and a small waist was associated with the lowest risk of heart disease. This benefit was noted in women of all sizes and seemed to mitigate much of the coronary risk typically associated with high BMI. For example, overweight and obese women (BMIs between 25.2 and 48.8) with large hips and small waists had a coronary heart disease risk that was only one-half that of women of about average, or slightly less than average, weight (BMIs between 22.2 and 25.2) who had small hips and large waists. *Body shape appeared to be far more telling than body weight.*

- Most recently a 2001 report on 695 men and women participating in the Quebec Family Study revealed that a large hip circumference was associated with high HDL-cholesterol and low triglycerides and insulin. The researchers emphasized the "independent" influence of hip size on cardiovascular disease risk factors and cited two other reports published in 1997 that found that "the total amount of fat in legs and hips was negatively correlated with risk of cardiovascular disease." *Again, the fatter the hips, the lower the risk of heart disease.*

What all these studies suggest is that a serious rethinking of our stance on body fat is in order. Never again can it be assumed that body fat is categorically unhealthy. There can be no meaningful statements made about body fat unless the location of that fat is taken into account.

The failure to consider location may help to explain why all the research on the health impact of obesity is so riddled with the kind of inconsistencies described in previous chapters. For example, *most* autopsy and angiographic studies show obesity to be unrelated to atherosclerosis. *Some* studies, however, show obesity to be an asset rather than a liability. In the latter studies it may have been the case that the obese men and women happened to have relatively larger amounts of *good* body fat compared with bad body fat.

It needs to be pointed out that the fat we are discussing here is *white* adipose tissue. There is also brown body fat, a very high burner of calories—hence an excellent generator of heat—which is plentiful on the bodies of infants and hibernating animals. Adults have relatively little of this type of fat (though there is some speculation that men and women who are predisposed to perpetual leanness may have a higher brown-fat-to-white-fat ratio than other adults). In general, however, adults mainly have white adipose tissue. The typical man or woman living in the United States has an average of about forty-five pounds of white body fat. White adipose tissue is of two types: "deep" and "subcu-taneous." All fat cells store fat.

Most of our body fat—somewhere between 70 and 80 percent for men, and more for women—is subcutaneous, that is, right beneath the skin. Body fat not stored subcutaneously is referred to as deep body fat, most of which is located deep within the abdominal area, around our internal organs, and is also called intra-abdominal, or visceral, fat. When there is a great deal of it, it may cause the entire abdominal region to swell, and result in the apple shape described above. Apple shapes can also result from large amounts of subcutaneous fat in this region, but usually they are associated with visceral fat, and it is that kind of fat that seems to be associated with virtually all health problems on which fat seems to have any bearing. Conversely, when there are large amounts of subcutaneous fat, as indicated mainly by large hip and thigh measurements, fat seems to perform certain protective functions.

Having established that some kinds of body fat are better than others, scientists have had to investigate what factors are involved in making body fat either good or bad; what determines which kind of fat we have; and what, if anything, can be done about the bad body fat.

Visceral (or Deep) Abdominal Fat: The *Bad* Body Fat

When Hippocrates asserted some twenty-four hundred years ago that "In all maladies, those who are fattest about the belly do best," he must have been referring to maladies other than the chronic, degenerative diseases that afflict modern-day industrialized nations. Those who are "fattest about the belly" definitely do *not* "do best" when it comes to such killers as heart disease, cancer, and diabetes, for example. This is due in part to the metabolic nature of visceral fat and its proximity to the liver—a crucial organ for the healthy processing of fat and carbohydrates.

Deep fat, unlike the other kind of fat, the "good" body fat, tends to be metabolically hyperactive, both synthesizing (taking in and storing) and breaking down (releasing) fat at a breakneck pace. One of the results of all this metabolic hyperactivity is that a considerable amount of fat is released into the bloodstream in the form of free fatty acids. Generally speaking, the more visceral fat you have, the higher the level of free fatty acids in your blood.

Some of the fat that is released can, via intricate and as yet not fully understood biochemical mechanisms, end up clogging your arteries. Because visceral fat is so near the liver, a lot of the fatty acids it releases go directly to that organ, which will be impaired in many of its functions if the fat levels in the bloodstream are too high. The resulting problems will be discussed in detail in Chapter 8. For now, suffice it to say that impaired liver function can result in high levels of insulin in the blood— a condition called hyperinsulinemia—which is one of the hallmarks of the metabolic disorder known as insulin resistance, which in turn is a forerunner of type 2 diabetes. High blood pressure, high overall choles-terol and low HDL cholesterol, high triglycerides, and poor glucose metabolism can all be caused by hyperinsulinemia. In short, a lot of visceral fat may bring about a big metabolic mess.

Basically three things determine how much *bad* body fat you have: genes, gender (men, because of hormonal differences, typically have about twice the amount of bad body fat as women), and lifestyle. Since lifestyle counts for a lot, and it's also the only one of the factors within our control, that's the one I'm going to focus on.

A Lifestyle Recipe for Bad Body Fat

If you want to create a lot of bad body fat, over and above that which is your destiny because of genes and gender, do the following: Exercise as little as possible, eat fiber-depleted foods loaded with fat (especially saturated fat) and refined sugar, drink a lot of alcohol, smoke cigarettes, and subject yourself to as much stress as possible. In other words, do as a great many Americans do. The effects of each of these behaviors are cumulative, so do them all for maximum effect. But if you can't indulge in every one of these behaviors, one or more will still be effective—especially if you choose physical inactivity and fat and sugar-laden food, the behaviors of choice for millions of Americans.

In Part Three, where I describe my Twenty/Twenty Program for Metabolic Fitness, there is a detailed explanation of how a sedentary lifestyle and an unhealthy diet create metabolic "unfitness," and of how *bad* body fat figures in this process. The abridged version of this explanation is that a lack of regular exercise tends to make the body lose its ability to burn fat—even visceral fat, which is the easiest fat to burn. Moreover, the two dietary ingredients most conducive to expanding the body's stores of visceral fat are fat and sugar, which constitute more than one-half of the calories consumed by the average sedentary American. So the poor diet and anemic exercise regimen of this typical American results in increased amounts of fat on the body and a decreased ability to burn it off.

High levels of physical exercise, however, seem able to counteract the accumulation of bad body fat—even in the face of massive calorie intake, apparently. This was the conclusion drawn by researchers at Osaka

University Medical School, who studied fifteen young professional Sumo wrestlers, with an average BMI of 36—way over the cutoff point for obesity by any standard—average daily consumption of 5,000 to 7,000 calories, and average exercise levels of several hours of hard physical activity per day. Despite their obvious obesity, the Sumo wrestlers had relatively little visceral body fat, as assessed by CAT scans. They also had the low levels of cholesterol (160 mg/dl) that seem to be associated with modest amounts of this kind of fat, as well as fairly normal levels of triglycerides (105 mg/dl) and blood glucose (95 mg/dl). The moral seems to be if you're going to eat a lot, then exercise a lot too. Very few people, however, will consume as many calories as the Sumo wrestlers, or exercise as many of them away.

How smoking and alcohol consumption figure in bad body fat is not fully understood, although recent studies have hinted that it may have something to do with their effects on steroid hormones, some of which play a role in regulating the size of visceral fat stores. Whatever the mechanism, there does seem to be a connection, which makes it particularly ironic that many people, especially women, smoke in an effort to keep their weight down. While smoking does seem to have the desired effect on body weight, it appears to work in the opposite direction on bad body fat, increasing rather than decreasing it.

Stress, too, plays a role that we are only now beginning to recognize and understand. Several groups of researchers in the United States and Sweden, for example, have done studies indicating that women with relatively large amounts of visceral fat—regardless of how much total body fat they have—are likelier to display high levels of anger, anxiety, and depression. While such observations do not prove a cause and effect relationship, animal studies have been done that do seem to demonstrate causality.

In a research program designed to study the effects of stress (and exercise) on body fat, scientists at Bowman Gray School of Medicine at Wake Forest University studied seventy-nine monkeys who were divided into two groups: a control group of unstressed monkeys, and another group in whom they induced stress by continually disrupting their social structure. Both groups of monkeys lived in groups of five, but the monkeys in the unstressed group remained in a stable, unchanging social environment, while the monkeys assigned to the stressed group were given new "roommates" each month. Monkeys don't like such arrangements, preferring life in a socially stable, fixed-membership club. They responded as predicted, becoming more aggressive, which is an outward sign of stress. CAT scan measurements of the two groups showed that the stressed monkeys accumulated more visceral fat, which prompted the researchers to conclude that stress itself may cause the expansion of bad body fat. Other health consequences in the stressed group included high blood pressure, elevated blood fats, and heart disease.

The critical link between visceral fat and stress appears to be cortisol, a hormone released by the adrenal gland. Under stress the adrenal gland pumps out large quantities of cortisol into the blood, where it has a potent effect on fat accumulation in the abdominal area. This effect is most visibly demonstrated in a medical condition called Cushing's syndrome, in which the adrenal gland pumps out massive amounts of cortisol. Individuals with this condition (which can be caused by either a tumor in the adrenal gland or a malfunction of the pituitary gland) invariably have a large amount of visceral fat and suffer from the accompanying health problems. When the condition is treated, cortisol levels can usually be normalized, with the result that visceral fat stores shrink.

Whether it's too little exercise or too much dietary fat and sugar, alcohol, cigarettes, and stress, it is apparent that as lifestyle goes, so goes bad body fat. This means that if you want to do something about visceral body fat and the risks that go with it, you've got to make some lifestyle changes—or hope that you have a lot of the good kind of body fat, for it may counteract the effects of bad body fat.

The problem is that good body fat and bad body fat are in a constant competition, with fat cells from both types trying to do their job, which is to serve as a repository for the fat that we eat. Which type will win the competition for any given molecule of fat is a complicated and incompletely understood issue, but it does seem that having a higher-than-usual ratio of subcutaneous fat to visceral fat can help—particularly if a lot of that subcutaneous fat is located in the hips and thighs.

Subcutaneous Fat:
The Good Body Fat

The hip and thigh fat cells have a ready-made edge in the competition because, not only are they vastly more numerous, they are biochemically better suited to taking fat out of the bloodstream. Unlike the fat cells above the waist, they are well endowed with a form of an enzyme (called lipoprotein lipase) that causes them to store fat easily and give it up very begrudgingly, to which most pear-shaped women will quickly attest. This is one of those good-news/bad-news situations: good because fat in the fat cells of the hips and thighs is believed to have a positive effect on health, rather than that in the visceral fat, where it can ultimately create a host of metabolic problems; bad in that it tends to *stay* in those fat cells, and our culture has taught us to want to get rid of it. (Hence the huge success some years ago of a little book called *Thin Thighs in 30 Days*.)

How do we know that we really should be rooting for the fat cells on our hips and thighs to win the competition, that there really is some as-yet-unknown, ideal ratio of good body fat to bad body fat that will make for better health? One test of this hypothesis would be to selectively remove fat from the hips and thighs and see what happens to various metabolic indicators of good health. Unfortunately no large-scale studies of this type have been done. On a small scale, however, there are a few studies that have examined the metabolic effects of removing subcutaneous fat. The first of these studies was performed in the mid-1970s by Dr. John Kral, a professor of surgery at the State University of New York Health Science Center at Brooklyn and an expert in obesity research. Dr. Kral did before-and-after health profiles on two women, twenty-nine and thirty-three years old, on whom he performed lipectomies (surgical removal of subcutaneous fat). In order to shrink their fat cells prior to the surgery, which would allow him to remove many more of them, he first put the women on diet and exercise programs that resulted in a drop in weight from 339 to 246 for one, 242 to 178 for the other, after which he cut away 13.5 pounds and 10.5 pounds of subcutaneous fat, respectively.

A variety of before-and-after tests were done on the women, including a simple lab test to measure the amount of triglycerides (fat) in the blood and a test to assess glucose metabolism efficiency. The latter, known as a glucose tolerance test, requires drinking a glucose solution and then, over the next three hours, measuring levels of glucose and insulin in the blood to see how sensitive the body is to this hormone. If relatively large amounts of insulin are present, that means the body requires a lot of insulin to do the job of metabolizing the glucose; in short the body has become insulin resistant, which puts it at increased risk for developing diabetes.

If body fat is unhealthy, then the last thing we would expect to see from these tests would be an increase in blood triglycerides and a poorer performance on the glucose tolerance test after the lipectomies. Yet this is precisely what happened. After the removal of what Dr. Kral estimated as between 12 and 15 billion subcutaneous fat cells from each woman, the women's bodies appeared less effective at getting fat out of the bloodstream, as indicated by the rise in blood triglycerides, and less efficient at processing glucose, as indicated by the rise in insulin levels. Although such evidence clearly lacks the impact of a large-scale study, the triglyceride test results are completely compatible with the findings of the researchers at Stanford and Laval universities, who showed an association between high levels of triglycerides and relatively low amounts of thigh fat. As for the higher levels of insulin after the surgery, those findings seem compatible with numerous studies showing a strong link between insulin levels and visceral fat. The hypothesis is that the reduction in good body fat after the lipectomy would have given the bad body fat the competitive edge, resulting in an expansion of visceral body fat stores, which then caused the insulin resistance.

The evidence here is only circumstantial, though. The postsurgical insulin resistance *suggests* that visceral body fat has increased, but doesn't prove it. By way of additional circumstantial evidence, Dr. Kral notes that in his experience extremely heavy women who have subcutaneous body fat surgically removed ultimately end up more apple- than pear-shaped, and they seem to have the health problems—high blood-fat levels, high blood pressure, diabetes, and so on—that go with apple shapes, unlike similarly heavy women who have retained their natural endowment of subcutaneous body fat. Though he postulates that such problems (and the apple shape that is characteristic of those who have them) may be due to a postsurgical expansion of bad body fat, no actual measures of postlipectomy visceral body fat have been done on humans.

Visceral body fat measures have been done on laboratory animals, however, and the results support the theory: Within a few months of the surgical removal of subcutaneous fat from the bodies of rats, the amount of fat stored in the abdominal area did increase. The visceral fat had indeed won the competition.

Since the seminal observations of Dr. Kral nearly a quarter century ago, surprisingly few studies—given the spectacular popularity of the procedure—have examined the metabolic effects of liposuction; the ones that have examined it contain mixed results. Liposuction is a sort of vacuuming technique, in which fat cells are literally sucked out of the body with a suction device. In one study, 53 patients with Dercum's disease (a disorder characterized by painful fatty tumors in adipose tissue) were evaluated before and for up to three months after liposuction. The fat removal procedure seemed to increase the risk of blood clots, which can cause heart attacks. Three months after liposuction, the concentration of a blood-clotting compound called plasminogen activator inhibitor–1, or PAI–1, was significantly elevated above preliposuction levels. High levels of PAI–1 are associated with high levels of visceral body fat.

On the other hand, one recently published pilot study concluded that liposuction might reduce the risk of cardiovascular disease. Fourteen overweight or obese women had an average of 13 pounds of fat removed, primarily from the hips, buttocks, thighs, and waist. In contrast to what Dr. Kral observed, insulin was reduced. However, glucose, cholesterol, and triglycerides were not affected. One puzzling finding was that four months after surgery significant reductions in fat mass were noted in areas of the body that were not suctioned, such as the arms. This raises the possibility that the women may have altered their diet and/or increased physical activity after the surgical procedure, and these changes may have been largely responsible for the improvement in fasting insulin levels. Indeed, the women continued to lose weight during the first four months after liposuction was performed.

What all this means for the hundreds of thousands of women and men (mainly women) who undergo liposuction each year is unclear. Because liposuction is a procedure done mainly for cosmetic reasons, not health, there have been no large-scale, long-term follow-up studies to determine if it poses a genuine "metabolic" health threat. The immediate surgical risks, on the other hand, are more quantifiable. Two independent surveys in the mid-to-late 1990s of physicians certified by the American Board of Plastic Surgery revealed a mortality rate from liposuction of about 20 deaths per 100,000 procedures. Compare this, for example, with the U.S. motor vehicle accident fatality rate of 16.4 deaths per 100,000 accidents. The American Society for Aesthetic Plastic Surgery reported 385,390 liposuction procedures in 2001. Since this figure represents a 118 percent increase from 1997, the number of procedures— and deaths—can only be expected to rise in years to come. As two physicians cautioned in a January 2000 report in *Plastic & Reconstructive Surgery*, "Liposuction is *not* trivial surgery, is *not* always benign, and is *not* quite as safe as intimated in glossy office brochures."

Remember, too, that if changes in diet and exercise regimens are not made, fat comes back. This occurs in one of two ways: Either your body forms new fat cells to replace the ones that were removed, or—the more likely scenario—the fat cells that remain in the body grow larger. For reasons we don't understand, visceral fat cells seem to become enlarged much more readily than subcutaneous fat cells. If it's the visceral fat cells that grow, that's bad news, because enlarged visceral fat cells seem particularly guilty—guiltier even than normal-sized visceral fat cells—of the kind of metabolic hyperactivity that disrupts normal healthy processing of fat and carbohydrates, with results that worsen the risk factors for cardiovascular disease and diabetes.

Are You an Apple or a Pear?

By now, you are probably wondering whether you are an apple or a pear; perhaps you're having trouble figuring out which one. This is because, while there are people with very large hips who really do resemble pears, and others with enormous bellies who really do look like apples, most of us have a body shape that doesn't match either fruit. Still, it is possible to determine, via the directions and diagrams provided below, which end of the body-shape spectrum you lean toward, and what that may mean in terms of the proportion of bad body fat to good body fat. This, in turn, may tell you something meaningful about your health.

First you have to take your measurements. (Keep in mind as you do this that body dimensions can be definitive without taking into account how you attained them, which has to do with your lifestyle.) The measurements are very simple, consisting only of waist and hip circumference; so, too, is the equipment for taking them: a tape measure.

Follow these steps:

1. Measure your waist while standing in a relaxed stance. No sucking in of the abdomen! This measurement should reflect the *largest* circumference around your belly, which will typically be at the level of your navel. If you have a substantial amount of fat around your midsection, sometimes the navel tends to be located beneath that point. If so, forget the navel as a landmark and just take the largest waist measurement.

2. Measure your hips. This measurement should be taken at the widest part of the hips, which is usually at about the level of the hip joint, or groin crease.

3. Divide the waist measurement by the hip measurement. This is your waist-to-hip ratio, which is a potentially meaningful indicator of your bad-body-fat/good-body-fat ratio.

Your waist measurement, considered in conjunction with the waist circumference diagrams below, helps to tell you how much bad body (visceral) fat you may have. However, since there can also be a lot of subcutaneous body fat around the midsection, an absolutely accurate measurement of visceral fat can only be achieved with expensive, high-tech medical procedures such as CAT scans or MRIs (Magnetic Resonance Imaging).

Your hip measurement, when plugged into a waist-to-hip ratio, gives you some idea of how much good body fat you may have. Though it may seem odd to measure the hip rather than the thigh, given the emphasis on thigh circumference in the studies mentioned earlier in the chapter, the reason is that the revelations about thigh fat are fairly new. All told, there are at least twenty-five times as many studies that use hip measurements rather than thigh measurements to assess the impact of body shape on health.

Once you have taken your measurements, use the following diagrams to assess your health risk. Keep in mind that for the most part, "risk" pertains to cardiovascular disease and type 2 diabetes. Whether there are other health risks associated with body fat location, we don't know, because the bulk of the research on body shape has focused on these diseases.

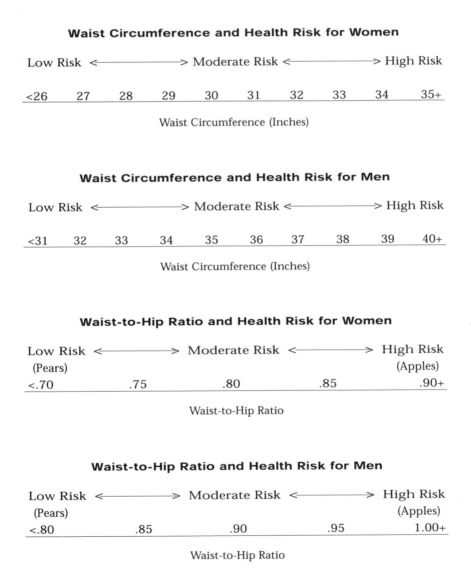

Waist Circumference and Health Risk for Women

Low Risk <————————> Moderate Risk <————————> High Risk

| <26 | 27 | 28 | 29 | 30 | 31 | 32 | 33 | 34 | 35+ |

Waist Circumference (Inches)

Waist Circumference and Health Risk for Men

Low Risk <————————> Moderate Risk <————————> High Risk

| <31 | 32 | 33 | 34 | 35 | 36 | 37 | 38 | 39 | 40+ |

Waist Circumference (Inches)

Waist-to-Hip Ratio and Health Risk for Women

Low Risk <————————> Moderate Risk <————————> High Risk
(Pears)   (Apples)

| <.70 | .75 | .80 | .85 | .90+ |

Waist-to-Hip Ratio

Waist-to-Hip Ratio and Health Risk for Men

Low Risk <————————> Moderate Risk <————————> High Risk
(Pears)   (Apples)

| <.80 | .85 | .90 | .95 | 1.00+ |

Waist-to-Hip Ratio

It may turn out that the two diagrams produce two different assessments of risk. For example, if you have a large waist but considerably larger hips, your health risk appears higher when using the waist measurement alone. On the other hand, if you have a small waist, but very slender hips, your health risk appears higher when using the waist-to-hip ratio. The way to resolve this dilemma is as follows: If your waist is in either the low risk range (below about 27 inches for women, 32 inches for men) or the very high risk range (exceeding about 35 inches for women or 40 inches for men) go with the waist measurement. The reasoning behind this advice is that people with waist measurements in the low-risk range probably have too little bad body fat, regardless of waist-to-hip ratios, to do them any harm. Conversely, for people with extremely large waists, the amount of bad body fat they have may be so great as to overpower their good body fat—again, regardless of their waist-to-hip ratios.

For all those people whose waist measurements fall somewhere in the middle, the waist-to-hip ratio is probably the best guide. In this context it's interesting to note that a twelve-year study of 1,462 Swedish women, ages thirty-eight to sixty at the beginning of the study, showed that the lowest risk for heart attack and death occurred in women in the lowest third of the waist-to-hip ratio index and the heaviest third of the BMI index (in other words, "large pears"). The highest risk was in the highest third of the waist-to-hip ratio, regardless of BMI (that is, "apples" of all sizes). A similar study on Swedish men showed the same thing.

How to Interpret Your Measurements

"Low risk" does not mean "no risk," and "high risk" does not mean that you should be buying a burial plot. Where you find yourself on these diagrams tells you nothing about your lifestyle, which must be considered before coming to any final conclusions about your risks. Body shape takes a backseat to lifestyle. For example, if your waist and hip measurements indicate low risk, but you eat a lot of fiber-depleted, fat- and sugar-laden food and live a sedentary life, then you should probably ignore the diagrams. In your case they give a false sense of security, and you need to think about changing your diet and your daily exercise habits. A pear-shaped or slender body is no guarantee of good health, and no excuse for being sedentary and eating an unhealthy diet.

Conversely, if none of the ingredients in the recipe for bad body fat are part of your lifestyle, and you still have a relatively large waist, and a waist-to-hip ratio that makes you more like an apple than a pear, then this probably indicates that your current body shape is natural for you, perhaps more a reflection of heredity than of anything else. (As noted above, it may also be that the apple shape is not attributable to large amounts of visceral fat, but to a lot of subcutaneous fat around the abdominal region.) If you're already living according to the recommendations in the Twenty/Twenty Program for Metabolic Fitness, and have no current health problems, then waist and hip measurements that signal high risk are giving you a false alarm.

Data from Aerobics Center Longitudinal Study (previously mentioned in Chapter 4) illustrate these scenarios perfectly, and reinforce the importance of fitness over tape measurements. In a 1999 report examining 21,925 men ages 30 to 83, the *highest* death rates were observed in unfit men whose waists measured less than 34 inches. In contrast, the *lowest* death rates were found in fit men whose waist measurement exceeded 39 inches (i.e., "fit apples"). It is worth mentioning again that "fit" in this study is defined very generously: all a man needs to do is score in the top 80 percent of his age group on a treadmill stress test.

Most people who fall into the high-risk area of the diagrams probably do belong there, however. If the recipe for bad body fat describes how you live, and you are more apple- than pear-shaped, then your measurements probably *are* a result of your lifestyle and, as such, an indication of being at risk for the diseases mentioned above. You *need* a healthier way of life and can find one in the Twenty/Twenty Program for Metabolic Fitness.

Despite the clinical distinction between good body fat and bad body fat, there can be no denying that the public perception of body fat, regardless of its location, is anything but positive. Most people lose weight because they view body fat as unsightly, in addition to being unhealthy. Cultural trends are hard to defy. And with a $30-to-$50 billion-a-year weight-loss business to urge them on, Americans find the temptation to diet almost irresistible. Perhaps some of the facts about the health risks of dieting, as presented in the next chapter, will help them to say no.

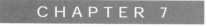

CHAPTER 7

Weight Loss for the Overweight and Obese:
Panacea or Pound-Foolish?

Dieting that causes excessive loss of weight...is beset with difficulties.
—Hippocrates, Aphorism 4, circa 400 BC

Until we have better data about the risks of being overweight and the benefits and risks of trying to lose weight, we should remember that the cure for obesity may be worse than the condition.
—Jerome P. Kassirer, M.D., and Marcia Angell, M.D., editors,
The New England Journal of Medicine, January 1, 1998

Twenty to twenty-five pounds. That, according to a telephone survey of nearly 108,000 adults that was conducted by the U.S. Centers for Disease Control and Prevention (the CDC) and state health departments, is how much 29 percent of the men, and 44 percent of the women, said they wanted to lose. Women wanted to lose more weight than men did (25 pounds *versus* 20 pounds), even though their average current weight was 44 pounds less than men. Regardless of the method used to achieve this goal—about 90 percent said they cut calories—few people come close to it. Men and women trying to lose weight typically report average losses of about ten to twelve pounds, and eight to nine pounds, respectively. It makes no difference how long they had been trying to lose weight. Actual weight loss almost always falls far short of goals and expectations. Despite our obsession with weight loss, data gathered from the four government-sponsored National Health and Nutrition Examination Surveys that have been done since the early 1960s (NHES I, and NHANES I, II, and III), along with data obtained from the annual Behavioral Risk Factor Surveillance System surveys, show that the average adult today weighs about 15-to-20 pounds more than men and women of the same age four decades ago.

The failure of dieting has not stopped us from trying it—over and over again. Nor has it dissuaded any major health organization from continuing to advocate weight loss to the estimated 118 million U.S. adults who, according to current BMI standards, are considered either overweight or obese.

What if these 118 million men and women were able to lose enough weight to conform to BMI recommendations? Would they then be in better health (health being the primary reason behind the public campaigns urging people to lose weight)? Countless studies have shown that weight loss improves blood pressure, lowers cholesterol, helps control diabetes, and so on. These are good things. Therefore weight loss must be good. This axiom has gone virtually unquestioned since 1918, shortly after the life insurance companies' initial warnings of the perils of "excess" weight catalyzed the explosive growth of the diet industry and helped make Dr. Lulu Hunt Peters's *Diet and Health, with Key to the Calories* this country's first best-selling diet book.

Evidence Refutes
the Weight-Loss Panacea

From the standpoint of health, however, there is a major problem with the "lose weight, live longer" equation: how to explain the two dozen or so studies published during the past 20 years that show weight loss to *increase* the risk of premature death, in some instances by several hundred percent. This is about twenty more than the number of studies published during the same period of time that showed weight loss to reduce death rates. Of the few studies in the minority, one showed an 11-hour increase in longevity per pound of weight lost—not exactly a ringing endorsement! (To gain a year of life at that rate, one would have to lose 796 pounds.) In two other studies, the reduced death rate associated with weight loss during the follow-up period was not observed in all subgroups of men and women examined; in fact, weight loss in some of the subgroups was actually predictive of a *higher* mortality rate.

The results can't be explained away as the product of extremes. None of these studies focused on drastic weight-loss attempts in massively obese people, or weight loss to the point of emaciation. The amount of weight loss associated with the higher mortality rates reported in these studies was, in most instances, between about ten and thirty pounds—amounts very similar to what dieters lose, or say they would like to lose, and what health professionals frequently recommend as reasonable weight-loss goals.

One of the most notable of these reports, a follow-up on the NHANES I study, which ran from 1971 through 1974, is a good example of how these studies are conducted. Dr. Elsie Pamuk and four of her colleagues at the CDC examined the possible connection between weight loss and death rates for 2,453 men and 2,739 women between the ages of forty-five and seventy-four, who had participated in that study. By 1987, 1,034 of the participants had died. Weight loss was defined as the difference between what participants reported to be the highest weight attained during their lifetime and what they actually weighed when examined by researchers in the early 1970s.

Dividing the men and women into groups according to how much weight they had lost, the CDC researchers put all those who had lost less than 5 percent of the highest body weight they had ever attained into one group; those who had lost between 5 and 14 percent of their maximum body weight into another group; and those who had lost 15 percent or more of their maximum body weight into a third group. The researchers then broke down the various causes of death and devised thirty-six different ways of comparing them, eighteen for men, eighteen for women. Mortality rates for the men who had lost over 5 percent of their body weight ranged from 40 to 180 percent higher than those who had lost less than 5 percent, in seven out of eighteen comparisons; for women the difference between the over and under 5 percent groups ranged between 40 and 260 percent higher for the "overs," in eight out of eighteen comparisons. In ten cases each for men and women, respectively, there was no statistically significant association between weight loss and death rate (although in fourteen of these instances there was a slight trend toward higher death rates associated with weight loss). That left *only one out of a total of thirty-six different comparisons* in which weight loss was found to be associated with a significantly *lower* death rate.

Unintentional Weight Loss Cannot Explain the Findings

The potential significance of this study, as well as the many other studies published during the past 20 years that showed similar results, has been downplayed by critics quick to point out that none of these studies adequately addressed one key question: What are the reasons for the weight loss? If the weight loss is involuntary, as many critics contend, the result not of dieting but of illness or of smoking, for example, then the higher mortality rates associated with weight loss don't tell us anything about the health consequences of dieting.

Interestingly enough, the American Cancer Society (ACS) did a major study, published in 1969, showing that weight loss increased the risk of premature death *regardless* of whether it was voluntary or involuntary. During the fall and winter of 1959-60, volunteers for the society began tracking the health status of over 800,000 men and women between the ages of forty and seventy-nine. At the time they agreed to participate in the study, the subjects were asked whether they had experienced any change in weight during the preceding five years, and if so, how much weight they had either gained or lost. Most importantly, those who said they had experienced a weight change were asked if the change had been intentional.

During the six years they were tracked, almost nineteen thousand of the participants died of coronary heart disease (CHD) or stroke. Whereas the study found no association between weight *gain* and mortality rates from heart disease or stroke, it found the reverse was true of weight *loss*. In twenty out of twenty-eight subgroups, as categorized by gender, body weight, amount of weight lost, and cause of death, *weight loss increased the death rate from heart disease and stroke* by anywhere from 7 to 167 percent. For example, if a woman who was between ten and fifteen pounds above average weight lost twenty pounds or more within the five years prior to the start of the study, her risk of dying from cardiovascular disease during the six years of follow-up was 167 percent *higher* than a woman equally above average weight who remained heavy, even though the new weight achieved by the woman who had dropped the pounds was right in line with height-weight table recommendations.

The authors of the report stated, "To our surprise, the relationship between change in weight within a period of five years and later death rates from CHD and stroke was about the same for subjects who tried to bring about the change as for those who did not try to do so." Since the study also found that people who were physically very active had much lower mortality rates than those who were sedentary, and that the benefits of exercise seemed only to increase as people got older, we can assume that those who intentionally lost weight and were therefore at increased risk of mortality must have lost their weight via dieting, rather than exercising.

Since that 1969 report from the American Cancer Society, only four studies of weight loss and mortality have distinguished between intentional and unintentional weight loss. One of these was a small study of nonsmoking older adults that offers limited insight. Although unintended weight loss was clearly more harmful than intended weight loss, it is not apparent from the data—the researchers reported no statistical analysis—whether intentional weight loss among overweight men and women altered mortality rates compared to overweight men and women who were either weight stable or had gained weight within the past year. Of the other three studies, all of which are large-scale, two come from the data collected during the earlier ACS study.

In the first, published in 1995, researchers from the ACS and the CDC focused on women between the ages of forty and sixty-four who had never smoked and who were overweight when the study began (and therefore might be expected to benefit from weight loss). Of the 43,457 women who met the criteria, 28,388 were classified as healthy, and 15,069 had at least one health condition that the researchers called "obesity-related" (such as high blood pressure, or a personal history of heart disease, stroke, or diabetes). Mortality statistics were assessed from the time the study began, in 1959-60, through 1972, thus adding six more years of follow-up to the original ACS study.

For the women with obesity-related health conditions, intentional weight loss in general seemed to be beneficial: Women who intentionally lost *any amount* of weight had premature death rates from all causes combined that were about 20 percent lower than women who experienced no change in weight. Oddly, the lower death rates were primarily due to reduction in mortality from cancer (30 to 50 percent reduction), not cardiovascular disease (despite the fact that the "obesity-related health conditions" diagnosed in these women mainly reflected cardiovascular problems). In fact, unintentional weight *gain* was associated with a reduction in cardiovascular disease mortality (6 percent) that was almost as great as the reduction (9 percent) associated with intentional weight loss of *any* amount. Overall, however, the results did suggest that for middle-aged women with health conditions frequently *associated* with obesity, intentional weight loss improves longevity prospects. Most important in this regard is the "good news" finding that the reduced death rates were independent of the amount of weight lost; that is, losing a few pounds was just as beneficial as losing twenty or more.

By contrast, among the two-thirds of the study participants who were healthy to begin with, intentional weight loss was anything but good. For example, compared with healthy, overweight women who remained weight stable, *women who intentionally lost between one and nineteen pounds over a period of a year or more had premature death rates from cancer, cardiovascular disease, and all causes that were increased by as much as 40 to 70 percent. U*nintentional weight *gain*, on the other hand, had no adverse effects on premature death rates for these nonsmoking, "overweight" women. These findings suggest that if you are overweight and have no health problems, you are probably better off staying at that weight (and not worrying if you gain a few pounds) rather than dieting to conform to some height-weight table "ideal."

In a second report on the original ACS data the same researchers examined the issue of intentionality of weight loss on mortality rates among 49,337 men ages forty to sixty-four (once again divided into those with, and those without, reported weight-related health conditions). These findings, published in 1999, were mostly similar to those observed for the women. For example, among the 36,280 overweight men with no reported health conditions, in no instance was intentional weight loss beneficial with regard to reducing mortality rate. To the contrary, intentional weight loss of between one and nineteen pounds over a period of a year or more was associated with a 43 percent *higher* risk of death from cardiovascular disease and a 48 percent *higher* risk of death from all causes combined.

As for the 13,057 overweight men with reported health conditions, results were mixed. Most significantly, and unlike the results for women, intentional weight loss was not associated with a lower death rate from all causes combined. In some instances the reverse was true. For example, compared to overweight men who did not change weight, intentional weight loss of at least 20 pounds over a period of a year or more was associated with a 13 percent *higher* all-cause mortality rate and an 18 percent *higher* cardiovascular disease mortality rate (even though most of the reported "health conditions" were of a cardiovascular nature, such as high blood pressure). The only apparent benefit of intentional weight loss was the lower mortality rate associated with diabetes—a roughly 30 to 40 percent reduction that was unrelated to the amount of weight lost. However, because deaths from this disease represented only about 12 percent of total deaths in this group of men (71 percent of deaths were attributable to cardiovascular disease alone), this had little impact on the overall results.

The only other research effort to evaluate intentionality of weight loss with regard to mortality rates is the Iowa Women's Health Study, initiated in 1986 with a cohort of nearly 42,000 women between the ages of 55 and 69. A report published in 1999 reflected data on 25,897 of the women who responded to questionnaires mailed out in 1992 and who were willing to provide information on lifetime weight-loss experiences. A total of 108 different statistical comparisons were reported, depending upon age, initial weight and health status, cause of death, and whether they had experienced an intentional or unintentional weight loss of at least 20 pounds. In no instance was intentional weight loss associated with a significantly lower mortality rate. To the contrary, trends in the data suggested the opposite. In 74 percent of the statistical comparisons intentional weight loss was associated with a *higher* mortality risk. For example, one might reasonably expect that overweight women would benefit from intentional weight loss. However, overweight women who intentionally lost 20 or more pounds had consistently higher mortality rates than equally overweight women who were comparatively weight stable. The results of this study suggest that overweight women might be better off staying that way: the all-cause mortality rate of overweight women was 5 to 10 percent *lower* than that of nonoverweight women!

As of 2001 these remain the only published data on weight loss and mortality that distinguished between intentional and unintentional weight loss. In most of the recent studies, however, researchers have gone to great lengths to reduce the chance that weight loss was a result either of disease or of smoking (which can affect weight, and is, of course, a factor in many health problems). Participants are carefully screened with regard to medical history to ensure that they are healthy when the study begins; frequently, deaths that occur relatively early in the follow-up period are not counted in the statistical analysis, in order to minimize the possibility that the numbers were skewed by apparently healthy participants who were enrolled in the study at a time when they had as-yet-undetected life-threatening illnesses. For example, in the CDC study described above, Dr. Pamuk and her colleagues excluded from their statistical analysis of the data all deaths that occurred within the first eight years of the follow-up period, and further analyzed their data separately for smokers and nonsmokers. Even with all these precautions, the result was the same: *Weight loss was associated with increased risk of premature death.*

Since weight loss is believed to be responsible for a reduction in many of the risk factors for heart disease—high blood pressure, cholesterol, triglycerides, and so on—Dr. Pamuk's findings about heart disease are particularly surprising. The highest death-rate/weight-loss association of all, for example, was for cardiovascular disease in women who were from average to 15 percent above average weight, who had lost 15 percent or more of their body weight. This would correspond to a weight loss of 22 pounds or more for a woman weighing 145 pounds. The result was a death rate 260 percent higher than for comparable women who remained "weight stable," that is, lost less than 5 percent of their total body weight. If that same woman lost only 5 to 14 percent of her weight—or 7 to 20 pounds—her mortality risk was 150 percent higher than if she remained weight stable.

Similar findings emerged in the Harvard Alumni study that was mentioned in Chapter 4, in which the positive association between reduced mortality and weight *gain*, when combined with a very physically active lifestyle, was reported. In a study of a subgroup, consisting of about 11,700 out of the original 17,000 men, Dr. Ralph Paffenbarger and his colleague Dr. I-Min Lee found that weight *loss* seemed to have the reverse effect: Compared with alumni who had weighed the same in 1977 as in 1962, men who experienced a weight loss of more than eleven pounds during that same period had a 75 percent greater risk of dying from heart disease by 1988 (though no greater risk of dying from cancer). This finding pertained in all weight categories, and was true for nonsmokers as well as smokers.

Perhaps the most powerful of all the studies to have found a connection between weight loss and higher mortality is the one done by Dr. Steven Blair (Director of Research at the Cooper Institute for Aerobics Research in Dallas) and four of his colleagues, which was published in the *Annals of Internal Medicine* in 1993. Over 10,500 men aged thirty-five to fifty-seven who were classified as being at high risk for heart disease were enrolled in the Multiple Risk Factor Intervention Trial in 1973. Generally speaking they were overweight and had high blood pressure and high cholesterol. Beginning in the mid-1970s they were weighed one to three times a year for six to seven years. By 1985, when the total mortality figures were compiled, the results were unequivocal: Weight loss, even for a group of men who would seem to be the optimum beneficiaries of a weight-loss intervention program, was dangerous. In the group as a whole, men who had a net loss of more than 5 percent of their body weight (about nine to ten pounds or more for most of these men) during the six- to seven-year period when weight was measured, had a mortality rate from cardiovascular disease that was 61 to 242 percent higher than men whose weights remained within 5 percent of their initial body weight. Among a subgroup of men who initially were up to about 20 pounds above average weight (BMIs between 26 and 29), a net weight loss of more than 5 percent of body weight during the follow-up period was associated with a cardiovascular disease mortality rate that was 195 percent *higher* than that of men with similar BMIs who did not lose weight. Weight *gain*, however, did *not* increase mortality from heart disease—neither in the group as a whole nor in any of a number of subclassifications of the group, such as nonsmokers, or men of a specific BMI.

The Weight-Loss Paradox:
Yo-Yoing to Death

What we have here is a paradox, with potentially calamitous consequences. Losing weight seems to increase the chances of dying from a disease for which weight loss is frequently prescribed to help cure! This brings to mind the most fundamental canon of all helping professions: "Above all else, do no harm." How is it possible for weight loss to be both therapeutic—in its effect on many of the risk factors for cardiovascular disease—and dangerous? The explanation lies in the fact that it is virtually impossible to discuss weight loss apart from weight gain. As the dieting phenomenon has grown, so has the average dieter's weight. Weight loss, especially by dieting, the most frequent means employed, begets weight gain; and, as Hippocrates cautioned some twenty-five centuries ago, is "beset with difficulties"—many of them almost certainly attributable to dieting's cyclical nature.

The weight cycling experiences of the Harvard graduates studied by Drs. Lee and Paffenbarger are revealing in this context. In 1988, when the most recent follow-up information was gathered, the alumni were asked how frequently they had dieted and how many times during their lifetime they had lost less than five, five, ten, twenty, or thirty or more pounds. When all the weight-loss attempts and total pounds lost were tallied, those alumni who had a *net* loss of more than eleven pounds between 1962 and 1977 actually had a *cumulative* weight loss of ninety-nine pounds—which means they had also gained a considerable amount of weight over the years! The health consequences of this yo-yoing were striking: Compared with men who maintained fairly stable body weights, those who had lost and gained the most total pounds had an 80 percent higher rate of heart disease, and a 123 percent higher rate of type 2 diabetes. Similar results were found for yo-yoers who had ended up with a net *gain* of more than eleven pounds—which suggests that it might not necessarily be the net gain *or* loss that is dangerous, but the yo-yoing itself. Indeed, those alumni who stated that they dieted frequently, or all the time, had nearly double the risk for type 2 diabetes, hypertension, and coronary heart disease compared with their former classmates who said they never dieted.

The higher rates of heart disease in those who yo-yoed the most have been found in a number of other recently published studies, including the Multiple Risk Factor Intervention Trial, just mentioned, and the Framingham Heart Study. After more than three decades of follow-up evaluations that included biannual body-weight measurements, those Framingham subjects whose body weights yo-yoed the most had up to a 100 percent greater risk of death from heart disease than those whose weights fluctuated the least! The 1991 report in the *New England Journal of Medicine* suggested, very tentatively, that these findings "raise the possibility that weight cycling by dietary means may have a role in the development of chronic disease." Indeed they do! But the traditionally conservative medical and scientific research communities are still holding back from any more definitive condemnation of yo-yoing.

So deeply ingrained are our ideas about the health hazards of obesity that they overshadow the apparently much greater health hazards of yo-yoing. Therefore health organizations like the National Task Force on the Prevention and Treatment of Obesity are still cautioning that the evidence on yo-yoing is still "not sufficiently compelling to override the potential benefits of moderate weight loss in significantly obese patients." Let's look at the implications of that advice. In Dr. Pamuk's study, women who were overweight (by BMI standards) and who lost weight in the moderate range (5 to 14 percent) experienced cardiovascular mortality rates that were 40 to 150 percent higher than overweight women who remained weight stable. It's hard to see what the "potential benefits" of weight loss were for these "obese" women! Indeed Dr. Pamuk and her colleagues questioned the conventional wisdom on weight loss in light of the increasing pressure on overweight persons to slim down: "The policy of recommending a return to 'ideal' weight to persons who are already overweight may need to be reconsidered. From the results shown here, this recommendation appears to be especially unwarranted for persons with BMIs between 26 and 29."

Lessons from Leningrad, Minnesota, and the Laboratory

There's nothing new in all this. On the contrary, the strongest evidence against yo-yoing comes from studies that were published several decades ago, when the seminal experiments implicating weight cycling as a health threat were conducted. By 1966 researchers had made such a powerful case concerning the hazards of yo-yoing that the U.S. government itself spoke out, in the form of a seventy-seven-page report on "Obesity and Health" issued by the Department of Health, Education and Welfare. Nine experts in health and nutrition used the report as a forum to warn the public that "the frequent weight gains and losses indulged in by many obese patients who practice what one writer calls the 'rhythm method of girth control' may be actually more harmful than maintenance of a steady weight at a high level." Justification for this conclusion stems from two kinds of evidence—one showing dangerous, potentially artery-clogging increases in cholesterol during the weight-regaining phase of the cycle and the other involving experiments on laboratory animals.

During the 1950s and 1960s, researchers were conducting animal experiments, not because they were interested in the consequences of what we now call yo-yo dieting, but because they wanted to assess the health effects of fasting, which was a popular method of weight loss at the time. With fasting being endorsed as a weight-loss method even by many physicians, these researchers were concerned—and with good reason. On the basis of evidence that had emerged during World War II, both from carefully designed studies and from the exigencies of wartime life, it appeared that food deprivation, whether it was intentional (as in rigorous dieting or fasting) or not (as in starvation) could have extremely serious health consequences.

The research done by Dr. Ancel Keys and his research team at the University of Minnesota has already been described in Chapter 1. In 1944 they put thirty-two conscientious objectors on a twenty-four-week diet, consisting of about half the calories the men were accustomed to consuming. During the weight-regaining phase of the Minnesota Experiments (as they were called), the researchers noted that many of the men seemed to be on the verge of congestive heart failure, with one man experiencing such severe cardiovascular problems that he had to be hospitalized.

A much larger study of the results of calorie deprivation—in this case unintentional—was provided courtesy of the German siege of Leningrad. For five months, beginning in October 1941, the German forces cut off food supplies to the city of Leningrad, thereby essentially putting the population on a semistarvation diet, at a calorie level similar to many of the diets still actively peddled to this day. Not surprisingly, people lost weight during this period, and hypertension was reduced, which certainly jibes with the common perception about weight and blood pressure. However, it's what happened after the siege was lifted, when food became more plentiful, that is surprising.

In the spring of 1943 Russian physicians examined ten thousand men and women of Leningrad and compared the results with a similar sampling from 1940. The incidence of high blood pressure had shot up by between 100 and 400 percent, depending on age. The rise of hypertension in the living was paralleled by a similar increase in the incidence of hypertension-related vascular damage detected at autopsy. At one hospital in Leningrad, during 1941 and early 1942, during the period of the siege, hypertensive disease was noted in less than 6 percent of the autopsies performed. By early 1944, more than a year after food supplies had been restored, that number had skyrocketed to 55 percent.

The findings reported by the Russian doctors in 1943 were so similar to observations made during the Minnesota Experiments that Dr. Keys and his colleagues were struck by the parallels. In 1948, they wrote in the *Journal of the American Medical Association* what may be considered the first twentieth-century warning about possible health hazards for the dieter, even one who has been advised by his doctor to go on a diet. It read, "Out of the Minnesota and Leningrad experiences grows the possibility that such a patient may be worse off, when he modifies or abandons his dietary restrictions, than he was before the treatment was instituted." Similarly, as the editors of the *New England Journal of Medicine* cautioned 50 years later, "The cure for obesity may be worse than the condition."

If a single cycle of losing and gaining weight can strain the cardiovascular system and damage blood vessels, what happens when a one-time episode becomes a recurring pattern? More damage. At least that is what a number of university research teams in the 1950s and 1960s found when they placed laboratory animals—mice, rats, dogs, and pigs—on a succession of diets that created a pattern of weight fluctuation resembling that of yo-yo dieters.

In one of these experiments, published in 1964, a team of veterinary scientists at the University of Illinois turned young pigs into yo-yoers by systematically altering the amount of food that the pigs were allowed to eat. Pigs were chosen as research "subjects" because they, like humans, are very susceptible to heart disease. Also, being an "all you can eat" kind of animal, pigs tend to be great bingers. Over periods ranging from sixteen months to nearly two and a half years, the pigs underwent anywhere from four to eight discrete "diets," each one consisting of a starvation fast followed by refeeding to restore body weight. Most of the fasts lasted about a week, with some going on for a month or two. After just a few episodes of yo-yoing, the pigs developed high blood pressure. By the end of the study the investigators detected severe damage to the heart muscle and coronary blood vessels of most of the pigs.

The researchers concluded, in no uncertain terms (unlike the hedging of many recent experts), "Aside from the obvious pertinence of such observations to the current popular recommendation by some physicians of repeated fasts for weight reduction...the observations appear to confirm previous suggestions of a basic relationship between starvation, refeeding diet and cardiovascular disease." This helps us to understand the puzzling findings of current epidemiologists, who keep reporting consistently higher cardiovascular disease rates in men and women who chronically fluctuate in weight.

Starvation (or fasting) is one thing, you may object, and dieting quite another—but it's apparently not necessary to go on a fast to do irreparable harm to the blood vessels. This was the conclusion reached by a study at the University of Mississippi School of Medicine, where researchers put laboratory mice on a one-time low-calorie diet. As soon as the mice were allowed to resume normal, unrestricted eating, their systolic blood pressures more than doubled within a week. Although the hypertension was transient, lasting just a couple of weeks, the damage was not. Researchers found evidence of coronary artery damage in 80 percent of the mice.

The results of these animal studies are entirely consistent with some of the more recent observations in humans. Recall from Chapter 3 the 1999 report by Italian researchers who found that weight cycling was associated with significantly higher blood pressures in obese women (147/90 mmHg in chronic dieters *versus* 125/79 mmHg in obese women with no history of dieting). Because the two groups of women were matched for a number of variables (age, socioeconomic status, physical activity level, nonsmoking, not taking any medications, lack of family history for hypertension, normal menstrual flow, normal glucose tolerance, and equal cholesterol levels), dieting history appeared to be the only difference between the groups that could explain the higher blood pressures.

In a more direct manner, German researchers made corroborating observations on 22 obese men and women who underwent 12 months of supervised weight-loss therapy (reduced caloric intake with or without the weight-loss drug Redux), and then returned three years later for follow-up measurements. Subjects in both groups lost an average of about 22 pounds during the first year, and gained virtually all the weight back during the three-year follow-up. Those having received the drug actually gained back an average of about 25 pounds, meaning they were worse off than before "therapy"—and in more ways than just with their weight. Systolic blood pressure was higher, as were triglycerides, cholesterol, and blood glucose. Taking the weight-loss drug during the first year, however, appeared to have nothing to do with the deterioration of cardiovascular risk factors during the follow-up—similar elevations in blood pressure, triglycerides, cholesterol, and glucose were observed in the men and women who dieted without Redux. For example, cholesterol levels increased by 25 mg/dl in both groups (from 235 mg/dl to 260 mg/dl in the diet-only group and from 212 mg/dl to 237 mg/dl in the diet-plus-drug group).

Chronic dieting can lead to cardiovascular disease in other, less obvious ways. For example, researchers at the University of California at Davis found that dieting depletes the body's levels of heart-healthy omega-3 fatty acids. After very low calorie dieting for up to five months, blood samples and adipose tissue biopsies from the initially obese women who volunteered for the study revealed a selective depletion from blood and body-fat stores of alpha-linolenic acid, an omega-3 fatty acid that is essential in our diet (meaning that the human body cannot make this fatty acid itself). Supplementation of the diet with a special formula containing alpha-linolenic acid during the weight-loss period did not prevent the loss of this important fatty acid. Because the typical American diet is relatively deficient in omega-3 fatty acids, particularly alpha-linolenic acid, it's entirely possible that the reduction in body stores of alpha-linolenic acid via calorie restriction may not be subsequently replaced when the dieter goes off the diet. The authors speculated that "a subtle but chronic risk state could be established if recurrent dieting depletes omega-3 reserves, and intake during maintenance or weight gain does not allow effective repletion." These findings offer one plausible explanation for the consistent epidemiological findings linking weight fluctuation to increased cardiovascular disease mortality.

The Low-Carbohydrate Way to Heart Disease

How to avoid the cardiovascular problems associated with yo-yoing seems obvious, if not easy: Don't regain the weight that has been lost. But that solution rests on the assumption that the health risks of dieting are caused only when weight is regained. Many diets can also cause damage even while the weight remains off. Consider one of the most popular weight-loss strategies of the past several decades: the low-carbohydrate diet.

This diet has a long history, dating back at least to the mid-1800s, when Dr. William Harvey, an English surgeon, prescribed a diet for one of his patients, William Banting, that was devoid of sweets and starches, but permitted unlimited quantities of meat. Banting was so pleased with the results that he popularized the diet in his 1862 *Letter on Corpulence, Addressed to the Public*. Variations of this diet surfaced over the years, but none to such spectacular success as was achieved by a spate of low-carbohydrate diet books a century later: *Calories Don't Count* (1961), *The Doctor's Quick Weight Loss Diet* (1967), and *Dr. Atkins' Diet Revolution: The High Calorie Way to Stay Thin Forever* (1972), to name but a few; each soared to number one on the best-seller charts. Although shunning carbohydrates to shed pounds fell out of favor in the 1980s, the low-carbohydrate diet experienced a sensational resurgence in 1990s, with *Dr. Atkins' "New" Diet Revolution* leading the way. *Protein Power, Sugar Busters! Cut Sugar to Trim Fat, The Carbohydrate Addict's Diet: The Lifelong Solution to Yo-Yo Dieting*, and *Suzanne Somers' Eat Great, Lose Weight*—again, just to mention a few—all soared to the top of the bestseller lists in the late 1990s.

Though most of these weight-loss plans were penned by physicians, they had unsuspected health consequences, which first came to light thanks to researchers at a number of institutions. In a study done by Harvard Medical School in association with Peter Bent Brigham Hospital in Boston, twelve young men and women who were hospital employees volunteered to try Dr. Irwin Stillman's plan in *The Doctor's Quick Weight Loss Diet*, which calls for 50 percent of the daily calorie intake to come from fat, 48 percent from protein, and a cholesterol consumption 4 times the recommended maximum. Even though their average weight dropped by about seven pounds during the period they remained on the diet (which ranged from three to seventeen days), the subjects saw their total blood cholesterol increase from an average of 215 mg/dl before the diet to 248, which placed them in the high-risk category for heart disease. (Their prediet level of 215 is about average for the U.S. population, but a little higher than the below-200 level that is recommended.) Most of the subjects complained of fatigue, mild nausea, and occasional diarrhea during the diet, and a few had to quit after just a few days because the symptoms interfered with their work. At the time the study was published, in 1974, more than 5 million copies of *The Doctor's Quick Weight Loss Diet* had been sold.

Another study, involving twenty-four obese men and women, focused on the diet plan according to *Dr. Atkins' Diet Revolution*, which calls for approximately two-thirds of the daily calories to come from fat, the rest from protein, and a cholesterol load nearly three times the recommended maximum. After eight weeks on the diet, the group's LDL cholesterol—the bad kind, which promotes fatty buildup in the arteries—had increased by an average of 19 percent. The ten women in the study had even worse results: Although they had lost an average of fifteen pounds, their LDL cholesterol shot up by 33 percent. Their pre-diet LDL cholesterol level of 119 mg/dl was in the normal range. After just eight weeks on the Atkins' diet, however, their LDL cholesterol rose to 158 mg/dl, which is just 2 points shy of the 160 mg/dl level considered "high risk." To make matters worse, their HDL cholesterol—the good kind, which fights fatty buildup in the arteries—had decreased by 10 percent. The book (and all its subsequent spin-off versions) whose diet plan delivered these results is still wildly popular and remains a multimillion selling sensation thirty years after its initial publication.

While such findings may seem irrelevant to long-term health considerations, since most people get sick of these diets within a few days or weeks and go off them, the facts suggest otherwise. Atherosclerosis is a disease characterized not by a slow, steady narrowing of the blood vessels over time but by *sudden spurts* in the growth of the fat- and cholesterol-loaded deposits that clog arteries. An abrupt increase in cholesterol level, or a worsening of the ratio between bad and good cholesterol, could conceivably cause such spurts. Just a couple of weeks of staying at a high-cholesterol count of 248 mg/dl, which was the level reached by the men and women on Dr. Stillman's diet, could do more harm than several years at a count of 215, the slightly higher-than-recommended level they were at prior to starting the diet.

Dieting Begets Bingeing, Which Begets...

Actually any diet, regardless of its composition, can provoke the artery-clogging process. This is because dieting frequently sets the stage for bingeing, particularly on foods that are not exactly what we would call heart-healthy. Intense cravings for foods laden with fat and sugar are common among dieters and are frequently mentioned by dieters as the primary reason for their failure to stick to a diet. In my experience, I have yet to meet a yo-yoer who went off a diet by grazing at a health food store.

No one knows precisely why dieting intensifies preferences for high-fat and sugar-loaded foods. Though there has been a lot of emphasis on the idea that the causes are cultural, having to do with the vast amounts of junk food advertising that are constantly beamed at us, there may also be a strong biological component. The fact that even laboratory rats develop strong preferences for fatty foods during the refeeding stage of a yo-yo cycle hints that the longing may be in our nature.

Worse news still comes from research done by Dr. Adam Drewnowski, professor of nutrition at the University of Michigan School of Public Health, which suggests that the more dieting a person does, the stronger the postdiet craving for foods high in fat and sugar. Since the mid-1980s Dr. Drewnowski has been searching for clues to what determines a person's taste preferences. With regard to dieting, he has found that those most likely to exhibit strong fat and sugar cravings are women of above-average weight with a history of large weight fluctuations due to chronic dieting.

The negative effects of bingeing are not limited to weight gain. Bingeing on sweet, high-fat foods after each failed weight-loss attempt subjects the dieter's blood vessels to the same kind of high-cholesterol stress described above, and that means the potential for an "atherosclerotic spurt," with all the heart disease risks that such a spurt entails. Over the long haul there are also other kinds of risks to bingeing. High-fat, high-sugar foods promote the gain of *bad* body fat, which, as explained in the preceding chapter, can wreak havoc with both your cardiovascular system and your ability to properly metabolize your foods. Heart disease, as well as insulin resistance and, further down the line, type 2 diabetes, are the possible results of such nutritional abuse of your body.

It must be acknowledged that dieting does not always promote bingeing. Nonetheless it is well documented that most dieters will eventually regain most, if not all, the weight they lost. So it is important to emphasize that no matter how fast—or slow—weight is regained following a period of caloric restriction, the health of the dieter may be at risk. Just one weight-loss/gain cycle can impair glucose metabolism and elevate cholesterol, triglycerides, and blood pressures, even if the weight regain takes up to four years.

Furthermore there is recent evidence that chronic weight fluctuation may lead to "permanent" decreases in HDL cholesterol in women. A report published in the November 2000 issue of the *Journal of the American College of Cardiology* concluded, "Weight cycling is associated with lower HDL cholesterol in women of a magnitude that is known to be associated with an increased risk of cardiac events as demonstrated in prior clinical trials." In this NIH-sponsored Women's Ischemia Syndrome Evaluation (WISE) study, 27 percent of the 485 participants were classified as weight cyclers (defined as a weight loss of at least 10 pounds at least 3 times). As a group their HDL cholesterol levels were 7 percent lower than noncyclers. Even more alarming was the fact that the HDL cholesterol levels decreased in proportion to how much total weight was lost during each cycle. For example, women who lost 50 or more pounds during each weight-loss attempt had HDL cholesterol levels that were 27 percent lower than noncyclers (41 mg/dl *versus* 56 mg/dl). A 1 mg/dl decrease in HDL cholesterol corresponds to a 3 percent increase in heart disease risk in women; thus the "extreme" weight cyclers had a heart disease risk 45 percent higher than that of noncyclers. The researchers also noted that the true adverse effect of yo-yoing might have been *underestimated* because the women who reported a history of weight cycling were significantly more physically active than noncyclers. Since exercise is known to *increase* HDL cholesterol, the data suggest that with regard to "good" cholesterol the adverse effect of weight cycling is more powerful than the beneficial effect of exercise.

Dieter's Dilemma:
The Risk-*versus*-Benefit Analysis

Even if dieting doesn't lead to hypertension, heart disease, or diabetes, the consequences of counting calories may be seen in a number of other ways. Take your bones, for example. Because heavy people are more likely than thin people to suffer from arthritis, dieting is almost universally recommended as a preventive measure. The rationale is straightforward: The heavier you are, the more stress you place on weight-bearing joints such as the knee and ankle. However, the fact that heavy people with arthritis also frequently have the disease in their wrists, for example, suggests that the connection between weight and arthritis is more complicated than we presently understand.

On the other hand, the connection between weight and osteoporosis seems much more direct. As reported in Chapter 4, there is ample evidence that weight, even at the overweight or obese levels, helps to prevent osteoporosis. Conversely, dieting seems to contribute to it. In a report published in 1993 by researchers at the University of California, San Diego, middle-aged men and women who dieted frequently had markedly lower bone mineral density, which increases the risk for osteoporosis, than those who had not dieted or lost weight during their forties and fifties. The more fragile bones in those who "stay on a diet" to control weight are probably attributable at least in part to the chronic state of undernutrition caused by most diets. It may also be due to weight cycling, according to more recent data on 169 premenopausal Finnish women. Women who reported a history of dieting-induced weight fluctuation had significantly lower bone mineral densities in the lower spine and forearms compared to women with no history of dieting (but who weighed the same as the weight cyclers).

It's estimated that osteoarthritis and osteoporosis each may afflict between twenty and forty million Americans. Choose your poison. Certainly, to improve quality of life, many heavy men and women with osteoarthritis may well benefit from weight loss. (It is worth noting that physical activity, even in the absence of weight loss, can improve quality of life in men and women with osteoarthritis.) But indiscriminate recommendations for all Americans exceeding arbitrary weight standards to go on diets to reduce the risk of wear and tear on their joints must be viewed with great skepticism. The risk to their bones may outweigh the risk to their joints.

There are many other risk-benefit analyses that have to be done in contemplating weight loss. Excessive thinness and a low body fat content can result in abnormally low levels of female sex hormones, for example, which play a role in optimal bone health and a much more obvious role in reproductive functions. With at least 15 percent of U.S. couples experiencing reproductive problems, we have to consider the possibility that dieting plays a role in our increasing incidence of infertility. Also, it doesn't have to be dieting that results in extreme thinness either. Even among women in the weight range considered healthy according to height-weight tables, weight loss by dieting can alter the normal function of the hypothalamus—the brain's "master gland," which exercises the ultimate control over reproductive hormones—and thereby affect fertility. This has been known since at least 1977, when a team of researchers from the National Institutes of Health reported in the *New England Journal of Medicine* that nineteen initially mildly overweight young women who had stopped menstruating as a result of dieting had experienced abnormal hypothalamic activity. The researchers concluded that the malfunctioning master gland was probably caused by the weight loss itself.

Gallbladder disease presents another dieter's dilemma. On the one hand, excess body weight is routinely acknowledged as a significant risk factor for gallstones. However, weight loss also increases the risk of gallstones. So does yo-yoing, as noted in one of the relatively recent reports from the ongoing Nurses' Health Study. This study, published in the March 16, 1999 issue of the *Annals of Internal Medicine*, was the first to simultaneously examine the effects of BMI, weight loss, weight gain, and weight cycling on the risk for cholecystectomy (surgical removal of the gallbladder). The results showed that weight loss and weight cycling significantly increased risk, but weight gain did not. Compared to "weight stable" women (defined as nondieters who never deviated more than 5 pounds from their current weight), one or more *intentional* weight losses of more than 5 pounds increased risk by 138 percent! Weight cycling increased risk by 31 percent to 68 percent, depending upon how many pounds were lost during the episode of intentional weight loss. For example, at least one weight-loss/regain cycle of 20 pounds or more (defined as severe cycling) increased a nurse's chances of requiring gallbladder surgery by 68 percent. These results are especially alarming given that more than one-half (54.9 percent) of the nurses participating in the study were classified as weight cyclers—a percentage that is not all that different from the general population. The fact that weight cyclers were significantly heavier than noncyclers suggests that the increased gallbladder disease risk commonly associated with high BMI may in part be due to the high prevalence of yo-yoing among overweight and obese women.

A potentially more serious dilemma for the female dieter stems from evidence linking dieting-induced weight fluctuation with breast and kidney cancer. In 1994, Swedish researchers found that two or more episodes of weight-loss/regain were associated with a 287 percent higher risk of kidney cancer in women. Data from recent studies on breast cancer in animals and humans also provide cause for concern. For example, researchers at the Barbara Ann Karmanos Cancer Institute at Wayne State University in Detroit reported in a 1997 issue of the journal *Nutrition and Cancer* that diet-induced weight fluctuation in female rats significantly increased mammary tissue levels of the chemical 5-Hydroxymethyl-2'-Deoxyuridine (or "5-OHmdU"), an established marker for DNA damage in cells. The relevance of these findings in animals comes from recent studies on humans showing that high levels of 5-OHmdU in mammary tissue and in blood are associated with increased risk of various cancers, including breast cancer. The Wayne State University researchers reported in 2001 that blood levels of 5-OHmdU were significantly higher in women whose breast biopsies indicated either precancerous tissue or invasive cancer, as compared to women whose breast biopsies were benign. The researchers summed up their findings by saying that "the mammary gland is adversely affected by chronic weight cycling" and that "cyclic dieting attempts at weight loss should not be viewed as a benign behavior in women and may be an important risk factor for breast cancer."

Nearly one-half of U.S. women are currently trying to lose weight—92 percent of them via some form of dieting. Both percentages reflect increasing trends over the past few decades. During approximately the same stretch of time breast cancer incidence rates in the United States have increased by about 40 percent. The breast is now the leading cancer site among U.S. women and the number one cause of cancer deaths among women between the ages of 40 and 59. Perhaps not coincidentally, dieting is most prevalent among women ages 40 to 59. All told, one in eight U.S. women will develop breast cancer in her lifetime, and one has to wonder how many of the nearly 200,000 new cases of breast cancer each year in the United States might be attributable in part to our obsession with weight loss.

Weight-loss drugs represent another significant health dilemma for those in pursuit of a slimmer body. Ever since thyroid extracts were first used to treat obesity, in 1893, a number of drugs, alone or in combination, have been introduced as "magic bullets" to assist the dieter. As with all drugs, effectiveness must be evaluated relative to risk. In the case of weight-loss drugs, none has come close to what might be hailed as the magic bullet. In general, "net" weight loss tends to be small, typically no more than about 5 to 10 pounds compared to those receiving a placebo, and this is in overweight or obese subjects initially weighing over 200 pounds. Moreover, the figure of 5 to 10 pounds undoubtedly overestimates the true effectiveness of the drugs, for two reasons. First, it reflects weight loss only in those subjects who completed the study; in some clinical trials dropout rates exceed 50 percent (weight loss among dropouts invariably is less than that observed in the subjects who complete the study). Second, most studies last less than a couple of years—and in several of these it is clear from the data that even the subjects taking the weight-loss drug show signs of regaining the weight they initially lost. Thus, a truly effective pharmaceutical for long-term (lifetime) weight management has yet to be documented. What *has* been documented, on the other hand, are the very real health risks associated with the use of many of the weight-loss drugs, particularly a few that have been extremely popular over the years.

The most high-profile example is the fen-phen fiasco of the late 1990s. The cardiovascular problems associated with fenfluramine (one-half of the fen-phen cocktail that was extremely popular in the

1990s until the FDA recalled the drug in September 1997) and dexfenfluramine (marketed as Redux and, because it is chemically almost identical to fenfluramine, also recalled by the FDA in 1997) have been well documented and highly publicized in the media. (For an excellent account of the fen-phen debacle, I suggest reading Alicia Mundy's 2001 book *Dispensing with the Truth: The Victims, the Drug Companies, and the Dramatic Story behind the Battle over Fen-Phen*.) These drugs can cause heart valve problems and, less commonly, the almost always-fatal primary pulmonary hypertension.

The health risks of two other weight-loss drugs—amphetamines and phenylpropanolamine—are also noteworthy. Amphetamines are potent central nervous system stimulants, and, due to their anorectic qualities, were first used to treat obesity in the late 1930s. Within 10 years two-thirds of patients treated for weight problems were prescribed amphetamines, and amphetamines continued to be a staple in obesity treatment for several decades, either alone or in combination with other drugs (the "rainbow pill" approach, so named because of the many different colors of pills). They ultimately lost appeal however, largely due to their serious side effects, which include increases in heart rate and blood pressure, cardiac arrhythmia, heart muscle damage, pulmonary hypertension, and stroke. Amphetamine use also has been linked to kidney cancer. The Swedish researchers who reported that yo-yo dieters had significantly increased risk of kidney cancer (mentioned above) also found that regular use of diet pills containing amphetamine was associated with a 306 percent higher risk of kidney cancer.

Approved by the FDA in 1979 as an over-the-counter drug, phenylpropanolamine became a common ingredient in appetite suppressants and in cold and cough medications. The drug is a central nervous system stimulant whose effects are similar to those of amphetamine; it can increase heart rate and blood pressure. Although its use in cold and cough remedies appears to pose at most a very modest health risk, phenylpropanolamine-containing weight-loss products may cause rather severe cardiovascular problems, especially for women. In the December 21, 2000 issue of the *New England Journal of Medicine*, lead researchers of the landmark Hemorrhagic Stroke Project, a multicenter study initiated in 1992 by Yale University researchers in collaboration with the FDA and manufacturers of phenylpropanolamine, reported that for women between the ages of 18 and 49 the use of appetite suppressants containing phenylpropanolamine was associated with a staggering *1,558 percent higher risk* of a hemorrhagic stroke! (Since no men in the study reported using appetite suppressants containing phenylpropanolamine, the risk for men could not be assessed.) The increased hemorrhagic stroke risk is most likely due to the drug's adverse effects on blood pressure, which increase the chances of a blood vessel in the brain rupturing. Because of this report the FDA issued a public health warning in November 2000 and, similar to its action with regard to fenfluramine and dexfenfluramine three years earlier, also asked manufacturers to voluntarily discontinue marketing products containing phenylpropanolamine. Nevertheless, phenylpropanolamine enjoyed a 21-year run as one of the most popular diet aids. The drug once ranked as the fifth most used drug in the United States, and at any given time in the late 1990s more than 9 million U.S. adults used over-the-counter diet pills containing phenylpropanolamine.

Eating disorders, particularly bulimia, are another possible consequence of our obsession with thinness and the chronic dieting it promotes. Many experts today view dieting as an intermediate stage between normal eating and eating disorders. One of these experts, Dr. Andrew Hill of Leeds University in Great Britain, recently questioned not just the health consequences but the very ethics of weight-loss practices: "Is the trade-off of reduced obesity but increased eating disorders acceptable or even morally justified? Self-imposed undernutrition in the cause of an externally appointed ideal weight may be a high price to pay for too many people." As noted in Chapter 1, some eight million Americans are said to be suffering from eating disorders, which makes for a great many people paying that price.

Who Pays the Price, and How High Is It?

Who are the people most likely to suffer the consequences of counting calories? That's easy: those stigmatized as "overweight" or "obese." The prevalence of dieting is directly proportional to body weight. According to the survey on dieting mentioned at the beginning of the chapter, between 35.7 and 70.1 percent of overweight and obese men and women said they were trying to lose weight—and the percentages increased directly with BMI. By contrast, only 8.6 percent of men and 28.7 percent of women in the so-called "normal" BMI range indicated that they were trying to lose weight. The prevalence of weight cycling, particularly severe weight cycling, and the use of weight-loss drugs, is also much greater among women and men with BMIs classified as overweight or obese. As mentioned in Chapter 3, because all of these facts are never considered in studies of the impact of body weight on longevity, the ubiquitous assertion that obesity *itself* kills some 300,000 Americans each year remains nothing more than a culturally biased assumption.

Though plenty has been said, in this chapter and those that precede it, about the possible health consequences of the cyclical weight loss and weight gain that is so typical of dieting, I'd like to leave you with one final and particularly grim account of the results of a weight-loss program. I'm not the first to use it to prove a point. Between 1980, when the results were first published, and 2002, this study has been cited more than 200 times in the scientific and medical literature—not as a warning *against* weight loss, but as proof of the health hazards of obesity, and the necessity *for* weight loss. There's more than one way to look at its results, however. As an example of how research can be used and perhaps misused in the service of the antiobesity campaign, this study is very instructive.

Between 1960 and 1975 two hundred extremely heavy young men took part in a weight-loss program at the Veterans Administration Wadsworth Medical Center in Los Angeles. The men fasted for periods ranging from a little less than a month to slightly more than two months, and each lost between sixty and ninety pounds. Over the next seven years or so, almost all of the men gained everything back, and more, and fifty of the men died—twenty-seven of them of cardiovascular disease. By contrast the mortality rates for men of similar age but of average weight would have resulted in the death of only four men. In other words, the obese dieters had a mortality rate roughly twelve times higher than average-weight men did. The authors of the study concluded that "no unusual factors other than obesity could have caused such extraordinary mortality." However, by the researchers' own admission the men, other than their large size, "had no acute health problems when first seen." That is, no health problems *before losing weight.* It was only *after* the radical weight-loss "treatment" that the men started having health problems: seventy-five developed diabetes, thirty-nine became hypertensive, nineteen were diagnosed with cardiovascular disease; quite a number obviously went undiagnosed, since twenty-seven died of it!

Twenty-four hundred years after he wrote it, Hippocrates' warning about the health hazards of dieting goes ignored. So, too, it seems, does that of Drs. Kassirer and Angell, as editors of the *New England Journal of Medicine*, which was delivered more recently. The physicians lamented that, despite the fact that "data linking overweight and death, as well as the data showing the beneficial effects of weight loss are limited, fragmentary, and often ambiguous," and "countless numbers of our daughters and increasingly many of our sons are suffering immeasurable torment in fruitless weight-loss schemes and scams, and some are losing their lives," losing weight remains the number one New Year's resolution and our national preoccupation. Caloric restriction is still almost universally recommended as therapeutic by health professionals, in spite of what Drs. Kassirer and Angell referred to as the "dark side" of our national preoccupation with dieting: a risk-*versus*-benefit analysis that is short on benefit and long on risk. More than a half-century's worth of research has produced a mountain of scientific evidence about the health hazards of chronic dieting and weight fluctuation. It now seems evident that in America today the real risks to health and longevity are more likely to come from dieting than from stable weights that are over and above those recommended by height-weight tables or BMI charts.

This, however, does not mean that you should monitor your weight every day and worry whenever it fluctuates by a few pounds or so. Small changes in weight are most likely the result of day-to-day changes in the water content of your body and are nothing to fret over. Those who are physically active—and therefore particularly likely to be healthy— are also particularly likely to experience these variations in weight, because sweating may cause them to lose several pounds of water, and sometimes it takes a while to "refill the tank." This kind of weight fluctuation should not be confused with that which stems from dieting. In any case the studies that implicate weight fluctuation as a health risk usually define "weight stable" as staying within about 5 percent of your average weight. This would mean, for example, about 7 pounds for a

135-pound person and about 9 pounds for a 175-pound person. Day-to-day variations smaller than those do not constitute "yo-yoing" and are not a threat to good health.

Actually, the ideal way to health would involve no monitoring of weight at all, and thus no dieting, and none of the repercussions of dieting. The solution to our century-long "failure" at dieting is in the Twenty/Twenty Program for Metabolic Fitness, which shows you how to eat a sound diet and live a physically active life so that you will be fit and healthy *at your natural weight*. The Twenty/Twenty Program—to borrow from another of Hippocrates' aphorisms—is designed to bring your body "only to a condition which will naturally continue unchanged, whatever that may be."

PART 3

THE TWENTY/ TWENTY PROGRAM FOR METABOLIC FITNESS

CHAPTER 8

Metabolic Fitness:
What It Means, How to Achieve It

Obesity may not be a direct cause of disease, but may serve as an imprecise marker for an imprudent lifestyle. Excessive consumption of alcohol, fat, and sugar, and inadequate exercise and dietary fiber all contribute to disease while promoting weight gain. If these lifestyle factors are the true culprits in obesity-related disease, then the current focus on weight reduction may be misplaced.

— Paul Ernsberger and Paul Haskew,
New England Journal of Medicine, 1986

The hope is that by using metabolic fitness as a measure of success, health professionals can shift the patient's focus from unrealistic, culturally imposed goals (for example, dress size or belt size), to the more appropriate and achievable goal of better health.

— L. Arthur Campfield, Francoise J. Smith, and Paul Burn,
Science, 1998

The fitness boom has been a bust, just like the dieting game. Surveys by the Centers for Disease Control and Prevention (CDC) in Atlanta indicate that about 29 percent of U.S. adults are completely sedentary, and an additional 37 percent are not active enough to gain any health benefits. How active is active enough, you may wonder. According to the U.S. surgeon general's report on Physical Activity and Health, released in 1996,

Americans are encouraged to accumulate 30 minutes or more of moderate-intensity physical activity on a regular, preferably daily, basis. Brisk walking at 3-to-4 miles per hour is a good example of moderate-intensity activity. Other examples are bicycling for pleasure or transportation, swimming at a moderate effort, golf (walking the course!), tennis, and mowing the lawn with a walk-behind power mower. Only about one-third of U.S. adults meet this standard—that's just for moderate-intensity activity.

If we instead use physical activity of a slightly more vigorous nature as the fitness standard, the kind that can produce significant cardiovascular benefits, only about 10 percent would qualify. According to the American College of Sports Medicine, the professional organization that established this more ambitious standard in 1998, that would require exercising a minimum of three days a week, accumulating between twenty and sixty minutes of physical activity per day, at a heart rate between 60 and 90 percent of your maximum, which is called the target heart rate. (A rough approximation of maximum heart rate is 220 minus your age in years. For a forty-year-old, that would mean a target heart-beat-per-minute rate of between 108 and 162, which is 180 multiplied by 0.6 and 0.9).

Most healthy, average-weight, middle-aged people could achieve the low end of this target heart-beat range with a brisk walk—at least three and a half miles per hour—or a slow jog. Think about it: A brisk walk for twenty to sixty minutes three times a week—sounds downright doable, doesn't it? However, because of our no-pain, no-gain mind-set, a notion that to be worth doing, exercise has to be hard—a notion that the fitness establishment has done a lot to popularize—many people don't think the low-end recommendations are worth following. Exercising at such minimal intensity barely feels like exercising. How could it do any good? So they push themselves into the higher end of the target range, find the whole experience difficult and unpleasant, and abandon it altogether. The health club membership gets canceled, the stationary bike is stashed in the basement, and the daily run is forgotten. They have missed the fitness bandwagon. Or, more likely, fallen off or been pushed off. If you feel like you, too, are one of these casualties, don't blame yourself. You're probably trying to follow a program that is too time-consuming, difficult, and ambitious to be realistic for most people; worse, you've been given all the wrong reasons to follow it.

Losing weight and reducing body fat, which are the central focuses of virtually every health and fitness book, should *not* be the goals of an exercise program (certainly not the primary goals). Health and fitness are the goals, as everyone would agree, but health and fitness cannot be measured by weight loss or fat reduction. Burn away 3,500 calories, we are told, and the reward will be a one-pound loss of body fat. Every diet and exercise book on the market gives a list of how many calories each exercise is worth. Consider the dilemma for the 44 percent of U.S. women who, according to the CDC, want to lose 25 pounds. At 3,500 calories per pound, that multiplies out to 87,500 that have to be burned off. Translated into calorie equivalents, for a 150-pound person to lose 25 pounds will require walking about 1,100 miles (at 80 calories per mile)— roughly the distance between New York City and Orlando, Florida. Now, that's one tough New Year's resolution. Is it any wonder that most give up even before getting to Philadelphia?

Fortunately there's no good reason to walk to Orlando, no reason to link health and fitness with body weight, no reason to measure success by numbers on a bathroom scale. There's a much more intelligent approach to fitness, which also happens to be much more realistic and feasible. It's called the Twenty/Twenty Program for Metabolic Fitness. The Twenty/Twenty Program is flexible, works regardless of your starting weight, allows you to be successful (and feel successful) regardless of whether you lose weight, and improves your health as soon as you begin it. For example, research shows that just one exercise session of the kind recommended in the Twenty/Twenty Program can release chemicals (endorphins) that boost your sense of well-being immediately afterward; can lower triglyceride levels for a period lasting several days; and can make your muscle cells more responsive to insulin (a benefit you'll understand better after reading the next section).

One warning about the Twenty/Twenty Program, however: You will have to leave all conventional notions of fitness behind. If you think it's impossible to be fit *and* fat; if your idea of exercise is burning a certain number of calories in order to lose a certain number of pounds; if you assume that for an exercise program to be any good, it will have to leave you drenched in sweat and panting for breath; if you are looking for a magical new weight-loss diet to follow for a few weeks in order to fit into that one-size-too-small bathing suit you bought in an overly optimistic moment, this is not the program for you. The Twenty/ Twenty Program may or may not result in weight loss, but that is not the goal. Something called metabolic fitness *is*. Everyone can achieve metabolic fitness, with a modest effort, regardless of weight, age, or genes.

What It Means to Be Metabolically Fit: Insulin Sensitivity

Metabolism can be defined as the sum of all the chemical processes, both good and bad, that go on in your body. Broadly speaking, being metabolically fit means having a metabolism that maximizes vitality and minimizes the risk of disease—particularly those diseases that are influenced by lifestyle, such as heart disease, type 2 diabetes, and cancer. It means living longer *and* living healthier, feeling like you are twenty-five when you are forty-five, forty-five when you are sixty-five.

Speaking more scientifically and precisely, metabolic fitness is mostly about insulin. Insulin is a hormone that enables your body to utilize the food you eat. It helps the body build protein, store fat, and regulate blood glucose (also known as blood sugar) levels. Without insulin you could not live, but too much insulin creates problems that can also be life threatening.

Consider the role insulin plays in glucose metabolism. Whenever you eat a meal with carbohydrates, for example, glucose (the primary carbohydrate your body uses for energy) levels in your blood will rise as a result of digestive and absorptive processes. Glucose circulates through the bloodstream, where most of the cells of your body will be unable to use it, until insulin arrives on the scene. This arrival is usually pretty prompt, as the presence of heightened levels of glucose in the blood is the signal to the pancreas to release the necessary amounts of insulin. Acting as a messenger, insulin then tells the cells in your body what to do with the glucose, and they, being "insulin-sensitive," do as they are told. Most of the glucose usually goes into storage—primarily in muscle and the liver—until such time as your body needs it for energy.

Sometimes, however, this whole process is thrown off by "insulin-resistant" cells (cells that don't "listen" to the insulin). As a result, insulin is unable to do its job effectively. Millions of adults—perhaps one quarter of the U.S. population—have cells that have become to some degree resistant, ranging from slightly hard of hearing to almost totally deaf. When insulin resistance develops, it doesn't affect all the cells in the body equally. Rather the cells that display the highest insulin resistance are those in the muscles and the liver, which happen to be the two most important organs in the body for processing glucose, and therefore controlling blood sugar levels. If these cells continue to be insulin resistant over the course of many years, the insulin resistance may eventually go on to develop into full-fledged, type 2 diabetes. This typically occurs only after a long, slow process of deterioration, which is why type 2, or adult-onset, diabetes is usually detected only in middle age or beyond. Recent studies, however, have shown that insulin resistance and type 2 diabetes are becoming increasingly more prevalent among children and teenagers.

During this sometimes-lifelong process, the body deals with the problem of insulin resistance by forcing the pancreas to pump more insulin into the bloodstream—the strategy being to bombard the cells with an overload of insulin and force them to respond to it. It's sort of like talking very loudly to a person who's hard of hearing. This helps, at least initially; but eventually, if insulin resistance continues uncorrected, it leads to a chronic overload of insulin in the bloodstream. Hyperinsulinemia, as this condition is called, is a double-edged sword. On the one hand, it helps to control blood glucose levels, which is good. On the other hand, it causes the cells in the muscles and liver to become even more insulin resistant, which is bad. The result is a vicious cycle: Insulin resistance begets hyperinsulinemia, which in turn creates even greater insulin resistance—and so forth and so on. Eventually the pancreas may become exhausted from years of overwork, to the point that it loses the capacity to release enough insulin into the bloodstream. If the insulin shortage is severe enough, blood glucose rises out of control and the end result is type 2 diabetes, a disease that afflicts about sixteen million Americans, mostly middle-aged and older.

However, that figure represents only the most extreme version of these metabolic problems. Research conducted at Stanford Medical Center and at Laval University in Canada suggests that insulin resistance is very common—that, as noted above, at least one-quarter of the adults in the United States may be insulin resistant and hyperinsulinemic without even realizing it. These conditions cause serious problems, even if they don't eventually result in diabetes.

Hyperinsulinemia can raise blood pressure, lower the level of HDL cholesterol in the blood, and increase the level of triglycerides—all of which increase the risk of cardiovascular disease. A number of studies published since 1979 have shown a strong link between hyperinsulinemia and heart disease. Hyperinsulinemia also makes blood much more susceptible to clotting, thereby increasing the risk of sudden artery blockage, which can lead to heart attack, stroke, and death. Abnormally high levels of insulin have also been linked to many types of cancer, because insulin is a growth-promoting hormone, which can stimulate the growth not just of healthy cells but of cancerous cells as well.

Are You Insulin Resistant?

Although there are a number of signals that indicate the probability of insulin resistance, the only way to be absolutely sure is to have one of several different kinds of laboratory tests. A simple blood test, taken after an overnight fast, can reveal whether your levels of glucose and insulin are in the normal range. High levels of either may mean that you are insulin resistant. Testing for blood insulin concentration has not yet become routine. By contrast blood glucose testing is relatively easy and inexpensive (fairly accurate glucose meters can be purchased at most pharmacies). A fasting blood glucose level of 110 milligrams per deciliter of blood (mg/dl) or greater may be indicative of insulin resistance; a level of 126 mg/dl or greater meets the American Diabetes Association's definition of diabetes. In that case your doctor may recommend a follow-up procedure known as the glucose tolerance test. This requires drinking a solution that contains 75 grams of glucose and having periodic blood samples drawn from a vein in your forearm for the next three hours. If you are insulin resistant, your blood insulin levels will be much higher than normal during the three hours your body is trying to process the glucose in your bloodstream.

"High-normal" blood pressure (systolic pressure greater than 130 mmHg, or diastolic pressure greater than 85 mmHg), blood triglyceride levels of 150 mg/dl or greater, and low levels of HDL cholesterol (less than 40 mg/dl for men; less than 50 mg/dl for women) also may be signs of insulin resistance, and in 2001 were officially recognized by the National Cholesterol Education Program Expert Panel on Detection, Evaluation, and Treatment of High Blood Cholesterol in Adults as risk factors for what is now more commonly referred to as the "metabolic syndrome." A plentiful amount of bad body fat is another of the possible indicators associated with insulin resistance and the one most easily measured at home, with no specialized equipment (as described in Chapter 6). If you have been leading a sedentary life and eating a high-fat, high-sugar, low-fiber diet for years, though, you should go to a doctor, not a tape measure, to find out the status of your insulin sensitivity (and, as noted above, your blood pressure and blood-fat levels).

Causes of Insulin Resistance: Genes and Beyond

The reason I make a behavior-linked recommendation for seeing a doctor is that there are several factors involved in insulin resistance besides the most commonly cited culprit, which is heredity. Genes certainly do play a role. Type 2 diabetes, for example, runs in families. Other factors over which the individual has no control may also contribute. Evidence from researchers in England, for example, suggests that impaired fetal growth may greatly increase the risk of developing insulin resistance and diabetes later on in life. The "small-baby syndrome," in which the fetus does not develop fully during pregnancy, may retard the development of crucial tissues in the pancreas and liver (organs that are vital to the healthy processing of glucose), as well as in the muscles.

Although the battle against insulin resistance may seem unwinnable due to heredity, we need to look at the other factors. Without question it is lifestyle, not genetics, that plays the biggest role in determining whether an individual who is genetically *susceptible* actually *develops* insulin resistance, hyperinsulinemia, or diabetes. Once again, as so often happens in the ever-evolving world of medical and scientific research, we can make a case for lifestyle over genetics with an example that was used for many years to make the reverse argument—that of the Pima Indians. The Pimas of Arizona are almost all insulin-resistant, and they have the highest prevalence of type 2 diabetes and obesity of any group of people in the world. As a result, researchers have long cited them as examples of the apparently inescapable influence of genes on obesity and diabetes.

That there is an *influence* at work here is undoubtedly correct. The Pimas seem to have a very strong genetic tendency—a legacy of the "thrifty gene" I mentioned in Chapter 1—to develop insulin resistance and hyperinsulinemia, and therefore to store fat more readily. Even so, to conclude that the Pimas are prisoners of their genes would be wrong, as we will see from a comparison of the Pimas of Arizona with a group of people from the same gene pool, the Pimas of Mexico, who live a life that is quite different from their Americanized "cousins."

In the United States most of the Pima Indians live on reservations near the Gila River, on the Sonoran plain of southern Arizona. Believed to be the descendants of Indians who migrated from Mexico more than two thousand years ago, the Pimas of Arizona created a sophisticated system of irrigation that enabled them to convert the Sonoran Desert into productive farmland and live off the crops—at least until Manifest Destiny brought the good life to a crashing halt. By the late 1800s white pioneer settlers had moved in, taken control of the land, and diverted the Pimas' water supplies for their own use, thus wiping out the Pima farms. The lifestyle of the Pimas then changed dramatically. With no farming to do, they became much less physically active; and their diet gradually became Americanized— which is to say it was high in fats and sugars, and low in grains and fiber. A few generations later they had the high levels of obesity and type 2 diabetes that made them famous in the annals of science. After all, since their levels were much higher than the rest of the U.S. population, even though their sedentary lifestyle and unhealthy diet were similar to that of millions of people in the United States, that seemed to indicate that the problem was all in their genes.

However, the discovery of another group of Pimas, who live a quite different life, has brought that conclusion into question. Within the past decade researchers working at the Clinical Diabetes and Nutrition Section of the National Institutes of Health in Phoenix, Arizona, have located a group of 861 Indians living in and around the village of Maycoba in the northwestern Mexican state of Sonora, who call themselves Pimas. Several lines of evidence—genetic, archeological, and anthropological—suggest that the Mexican Pimas are indeed related to the Arizona Pimas. Unlike their American counterparts, the Pimas living in the village of Maycoba still lead a very agrarian existence, working in the fields several hours a day and consuming a relatively low-fat, high-fiber diet. Also unlike their American counterparts, who have a similar, if not identical, genetic heritage, the Pimas have a very low rate of type 2 diabetes and are rarely obese, their weights averaging thirty-five to fifty-five pounds less.

What this must mean is that genetics plays only a permissive role. It *allows* the genetically susceptible to become insulin resistant, obese, and diabetic; it doesn't *cause* them to. As the Pimas of Maycoba prove, genetic destiny can be kept in check with the right kind of lifestyle.

What would happen if the Pimas of Maycoba suddenly switched to a more Americanized way of life? Chances are they would become like the Pimas of Arizona. This is only a hypothesis, of course, but when comparable changes occurred in other populations who formerly had a healthier lifestyle, health problems of the kind associated with insulin resistance did result. Researchers working with the Tarahumara Indians of Mexico and the Aborigines of Australia have reported the negative results that occurred when these peoples switched from their typical low-fat, high-starch, and high-fiber diet to one that more closely resembled that of the typical American. Cross-cultural studies of Chinese and Japanese emigrants to the United States who adopted our lifestyle show that they, too, are fatter and have higher rates of heart disease and diabetes than their fellow countrymen and countrywomen back home, who consume diets with only about half the amount of fat.

One Recipe, Two Results: Insulin Resistance and Bad Body Fat

The lifestyle factors that are most influential in creating the insulin resistance syndrome are very similar to the ingredients in the recipe for bad body fat, as described in Chapter 6: lack of physical activity, a diet high in fat and sugar and low in fiber, smoking, and stress—especially the first two on the list. However, none of these is the lifestyle factor most usually cited. That distinction belongs to weight—to excess weight, that is. Since around nine out of ten people with type 2 diabetes—the ultimate outcome of insulin resistance—

are indeed medically classifiable as overweight or obese, it does seem plausible that weight is the problem.

If that were true, though, then reducing to a nonoverweight condition would be the necessary cure. As explained in Chapter 3, the health problems associated with insulin resistance—type 2 diabetes, hypertension, high blood cholesterol and triglycerides—can all be remedied without conforming to weight guidelines of any kind, even by those who remain significantly obese. Conversely, weight-loss diets such as the low-carbohydrate plans that have been so popular over the years, and have indeed resulted (however briefly) in impressive weight reductions, do not cause these problems to go away and may worsen them significantly (see Chapter 7). A recent critical review and computer analysis of all weight-reducing diets concluded: "While high-fat diets may promote short-term weight loss, the potential hazards for worsening risk for progression of atherosclerosis override the short-term benefits. Individuals derive the greatest health benefits from diets low in saturated fat and high in carbohydrate and fiber: these increase sensitivity to insulin and lower risk for CHD."

Being fat is not the problem. As mentioned at the outset of this chapter, body fat, or having gained a lot of it, is perhaps best viewed as an "imprecise marker for an imprudent lifestyle." The two primary causes of insulin resistance are a sedentary lifestyle and a high-fat, high-sugar, and low-fiber diet, which are also the two biggest factors in gaining weight (especially in those with the strongest genetic tendency to fat-storage-expansion—those with the "thriftiest" genes).

This is another of those health situations in which a vicious cycle gets activated, because hyperinsulinemia, which is the inevitable accompaniment to insulin resistance, creates a metabolic situation quite conducive to getting fat. The reason for this is that insulin is a very powerful stimulator for fat storage. The more insulin there is in the bloodstream, the greater the likelihood that the body will operate in a fat-storing mode (as evidenced by the observation that insulin therapy in people with diabetes routinely results in weight gain). Thus, even if a person doesn't eat too much, he is likely to keep getting fatter if he is insulin resistant. Over the years it may take for that same person to ultimately develop diabetes, he will probably gain a lot of weight, mostly in the form of fat, which explains why those with type 2 diabetes are usually fat.

Take away the insulin resistance, however, which the Twenty/Twenty Program is designed to do, and the type 2 diabetic condition is greatly improved, if not "cured," even if the person remains fat.

The Twenty/Twenty Program for Metabolic Fitness

The program I have developed has two key features: an average of 20 minutes per day of physical activity and a food plan with approximately 20 percent of the daily calories coming from fat. Twenty minutes per day of exercise is considered by most experts to be the minimum amount of time necessary to bring about improvements in metabolic fitness. Even this recommendation has some flexibility to it, since the twenty minutes per day is an *average*, not an absolute. The goal is at least 140 minutes a week of physical activity (20 minutes times seven days), which can be packaged any way you like—35 to 45 minutes three or four times a week; 20 minutes a day; or a mix of many short 5- to 10-minute activities and a few longer ones lasting 20, 30, or 60 minutes. I'll give you some tips on how to achieve this in the next chapter. You'll be surprised to find that many activities you probably never thought of as exercise can be thrown into this mix.

The 20 percent fat-content recommendation is based on my evaluation of the scientific evidence. The key piece of scientific evidence is the fact that our stone-age ancestors consumed about 20 percent of their calories as fat, and that seems to be the level of fat intake for which our bodies were designed. Although most public health organizations are currently recommending levels of fat intake up to 30 percent—perhaps because 30 percent is a significant improvement over the roughly 35 percent level that the average American consumes—that is *not* the optimum level for good health. At 30 percent the diet is still too high in fat to help minimize the risks of heart disease, diabetes, and cancer. Twenty percent is a better figure to aim for, even if you don't achieve it.

With only 10 to 15 percent of Americans eating a diet that falls below the 30 percent fat level, it may seem that the 20 percent level is just not feasible. Who cares what people in the Stone Age ate, after all? Presumably they ate what they ate because it was what was available, not because it was healthy or delicious. We don't have to look back into prehistory to find examples of people who eat diets of the kind I am recommending, however. Roughly two-thirds of the world now consumes a diet with a fat content of 25 percent or less, including affluent countries such as Japan, where there can be no question about whether the diet is one of deprivation or choice. Keep in mind, too, that the 20 percent figure is, like the 20-minute figure, an average. Splurging on high-fat foods such as ice cream is not taboo, and no foods are off limits. It's just that the high-fat ones have to be counterbalanced by low- or no-fat foods (especially those packed with fiber), so that the total comes out to *about* 20 percent. In Chapter 10 I'll show you how to achieve this balancing act so that you get to eat the foods you like while still keeping close to the 20 percent target. You will be able to create a food plan that will keep you fit, healthy, and feeling satisfied.

One of the best features of this plan is that the exercise and nutrition components work independently of each other. Since the effects are additive, doing both is optimal. But doing either one of them will still improve metabolic fitness and, as a result, your overall health, by increasing insulin sensitivity and thereby reducing blood insulin levels. Doing either or both incompletely—exercising 10 or 15 minutes a day, for example, or eating 25 or 30 percent of your calories as fat—is still helpful. Every little bit helps, especially if you are starting from a completely sedentary way of life and from a very high-fat diet. The farther away you are from a healthy lifestyle, the more every change you make counts.

I designed this to be a failure-free program, a plan that makes you feel that any part of it you manage to follow to any degree makes you a success. Unlike the plans that are supposed to get you to some ideal body weight that you either never achieve or never maintain, this one puts you at peace with your body. You may never again weigh what you did in your twenties, may never look like the models in the ads, and may never conform to any of the height-weight-table or BMI chart recommendations that your doctor keeps holding up to you. But you can achieve a natural, healthy body weight that is right for you.

Metabolic Fitness, Insulin Resistance, and Weight

I am a realist and acknowledge that in a weight-obsessed country like ours, most people will inevitably ask the question: Will I lose any? The answer is, "Probably," if you've been eating a typical American diet and not exercising. This will happen even though weight loss is not the goal of the program, only a side effect of a healthy lifestyle.

Just how much weight you might lose will depend on how far you currently are from your natural, healthy weight, and how much of the Twenty/Twenty Program you follow. I have known people who lost nothing more than a couple of pounds, and others who have lost more than 100 pounds, and kept it off for years. The major difference between them was that the former were probably already close to the weight that was right for them.

Even if you don't lose much weight, you will almost certainly lose some bad body fat—the kind that results from an unhealthy lifestyle and that contributes to many of the risk factors for poor health. But bad body fat represents only a small percentage of your body weight, typically making up less than ten pounds of the total in the average adult man or woman.

Keep in mind that no matter how healthy your new lifestyle, chances are that if you are middle-aged or older, you won't be losing *all* the bad body fat or all the weight that you've put on over the years. As explained in Chapter 5, the weight you gained is probably mostly fat, and once you've got them, your fat cells are yours for life. You can shrink them, but only so much, the amount varying from person to person. So how much weight you might lose is just not possible to predict with any degree of certainty, and it may not be the amount you are hoping for. Nor will you necessarily regain the same level of insulin sensitivity you had when you were in your teens or twenties. Sometimes it's simply not possible to totally undo a lifetime's worth of unhealthy living—though it's a lot more probable that you will regain most of your original insulin sensitivity than that you will lose most of the pounds you have put on with age.

What you will definitely be able to do on the Twenty/Twenty Program is to reverse a lot of the damage you've done to your body, and achieve significant improvements in metabolic fitness. As for weight loss—you will find your own natural, healthy weight, but without actually looking for it.

As much as most people want to lose weight, you may also be wondering, in light of some of the information in Chapter 7 about weight loss as a health risk, how I can advocate a lifestyle program that may well produce that result. Not to worry. The evidence regarding exercise and a low-fat, high-fiber dietary regimen is overwhelmingly positive. Also, most of the ill effects of any intentional weight loss are probably due to yo-yoing, not to weight loss itself. The Twenty/Twenty Program won't lead to yo-yoing because it is not a diet or a temporary plan for achieving short-range goals, but a lifetime, lifestyle plan that is intended to lead to permanent changes of a kind that will improve health and increase longevity. If weight loss is a side effect of achieving that goal, and weight loss is what you want, so much the better!

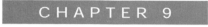

CHAPTER 9

Exercise for Metabolic Fitness:
Shaping Up without Necessarily Changing Shape

Healthy bodies come in all shapes. We need to stop hounding people about their weight and encourage them to eat a healthful diet and exercise.

—Dr. Steven Blair, Director of Research at the Cooper Institute for Aerobics Research; *The Walking Magazine*, 1995.

Before you read any farther, stop. Put down this book and take a two-minute walk, unless you already consider yourself a regular exerciser, in which case you can skip the walk and probably the chapter, as well. But if you are like most Americans, who, whenever they get the urge to exercise, take George Bernard Shaw's advice and "lie down on the sofa until it goes away," then stop right here and take that two-minute walk. Don't worry about the pace; it can be casual or brisk; right now, the intensity doesn't matter. It doesn't matter where you do it, indoors or outdoors, around your living room or up and down the stairs. Just do it.

You have started your exercise program.

I know, it sounds ridiculous. However, given that 40 percent of U.S. men and women over the age of seventy-five—5 million people in all—have difficulty walking one-quarter mile, it's not so ridiculous. True, one two-minute walk does not add up to a fitness program, but it's a start. It also gets you past the greatest obstacle to becoming more physically active: inertia, which *Webster's* defines as "an indisposition to motion, exertion, or change." Sounds like your average couch potato, the remote in one hand, chips in the other, doesn't it?

Overcoming inertia must come from within. My experience with exercise tells me that that's a lot likelier if the initial effort is quick, simple, and as painless as possible. That's why I didn't suggest a sixty-minute walk, or even a twenty-minute walk. Why two minutes? I got the idea from Dr. Steven Blair, Director of Research at the Cooper Institute for Aerobics Research in Dallas. One of the world's foremost researchers on the health benefits of exercise, Dr. Blair is also the senior scientific editor of the first Surgeon General's Report on Physical Activity and Health, released in the spring of 1996, and coauthor of a book called *Active Living Every Day*. Dr. Blair suggests a two-minute walk as a great way to get started, particularly for the inertia-afflicted who protest "I just don't have the time or energy." Everyone has two minutes to spare, and everyone has enough energy for a two-minute walk.

So do it. Then think about how you can incorporate several two-minute walks into your day—just by making simple changes in your routine, such as looking for the farthest, rather than the closest, parking space at the grocery store. Pretty soon the minutes start adding up, until you've got twenty minutes or so per day, for a total of at least 140 minutes a week.

"Exercise Lite"
for Metabolic Fitness

This is not a traditional exercise program, but we now understand that improved health, insofar as it relates to reduced risk of developing the insulin resistance syndrome and the serious diseases associated with it—diseases that are now this country's biggest killers—does not require a traditional type of program. The multiple two-minute-walk approach, though it is a considerable departure from exercise standards established in previous years, *is* consistent with the very latest recommendations made by the U.S. government and the American College of Sports Medicine (ACSM), which is the foremost organization of sports medicine professionals in the world. As described in the 1996 U.S. Surgeon General's report on Physical Activity and Health, the new-wave approach to exercise places a premium on nonvigorous, no-sweat-required physical activity. Many activities that never made the grade as "aerobic" now qualify as worth doing. When launched in the mid-1990s, the ACSM and CDC called the new approach "Exercise Lite."

The primary goal of the new physical activity guidelines is a reduction in the estimated 250,000 deaths a year attributable to lack of regular physical activity—deaths caused mainly by heart disease, cancer, and type 2 diabetes. The official position is to inspire Americans to accumulate 30 minutes or more of moderate-intensity physical activity on most, preferably all, days of the week. Since "most" could be construed to mean "more than half," that is, four days a week, the range they are recommending is somewhere between four and seven days of exercise, for a total of 120 to 210 minutes, per week. The 140 minutes I am recommending is within their guidelines, but at the lower end of the range for time commitment.

The major change from existing guidelines was a new focus on "physical activity" rather than "exercise," with much less emphasis on a planned, structured program of continuous, rhythmical movement at a relatively high intensity—vigorous aerobic exercise, in short—and more emphasis on just trying to get moving, at *any* intensity. The new recommendations no longer required exercise sessions of a certain length, but allowed for the accumulation of many short periods of activity throughout the day—a few minutes here, a few minutes there, and so forth. Hence the two-minute walk suggestion.

Yard work, household chores, home repair, fishing, golfing, racket sports, horseback riding, softball, skiing, volleyball, basketball, football, soccer, and even playing actively with children, to name a few—some vigorous, some not—now count. Experts now feel that the traditional fitness prescription was too narrowly defined, too demanding, too unrealistic. Now you don't need special clothes, and you don't have to go to a track or swimming pool or gym or fitness center. For all of you who don't want to or can't take part in those kinds of exercise programs, Exercise Lite focuses on spontaneous, unstructured activity—activity that occurs as a natural part of daily life rather than during a time set aside for the dreaded "workout." Think about how children exercise. Every day they go out and *play* (or at least those who aren't too glued to the computer or the television do). When was the last time one of the neighborhood children knocked on your door to ask if your son or daughter could come out and "exercise"?

Unfortunately grownups don't play enough anymore, and all of our modern conveniences have come close to eliminating the need for any physical activity whatsoever. Every now and again we may think about trying to go on a fitness program, generally involving a workout defined by parameters of time, frequency, intensity, and, most important of all, calorie burnoff. But the very word *workout* says everything you need to know about why few of us keep to a regular fitness schedule. Who wants to do a "workout" on top of a full day of work? You won't have to with these new guidelines, and you *will* be able to use them to develop *metabolic* fitness.

The new approach does not replace existing guidelines for developing and maintaining *cardiorespiratory* fitness—a measure of fitness officially defined by numbers indicating the maximum amount of oxygen you are able to use per minute, per kilogram of body weight, during an exercise stress test, which is usually done on a treadmill or exercise bike. The harder you are able to work—the longer, farther, and faster you can go—the more oxygen you will be able to use and the better your score. How well your body is able to deliver oxygen from the lungs to the muscles, which is what cardiorespiratory or aerobic fitness is all about, is one kind of fitness, but it's not the only kind. Although it is definitely the kind that has gotten almost all the attention in recent decades, it's probably not the most important kind in terms of health and longevity, and it's definitely not the kind over which you have the most control. Metabolic fitness is.

Metabolic Fitness *versus* Cardiorespiratory Fitness: Being Active *versus* Being "Fit"

Findings from the Copenhagen Male Study show the importance of just being physically active, as opposed to being cardiorespiratorially fit. Researchers at the State University Hospital of Copenhagen tracked

4,999 Danish men between the ages of forty and fifty-nine from 1970 to 1988. All the men were given exercise stress tests to determine their cardiorespiratory fitness, and on the basis of those results they were assigned to one of five levels of fitness. All of the men also filled in questionnaires about their activity levels. Based on their self-descriptions, they were classified as either sedentary (those who performed almost no physical activity and spent most of their leisure time reading, watching TV, going to movies, and so forth); medium active (those who spent several hours a week doing activities ranging from light gardening to table tennis or bowling); or very active (those who spent a number of hours each week in such vigorous activities as running, swimming, and tennis). In general, the sedentary men had a 70 percent higher mortality rate from heart disease than the active men, *regardless of activity level*, because mortality rates did not differ between those who were medium active and those who were very active. This suggests that it is not necessary to engage in vigorous activity to reap the health benefits of exercise. Simply being physically active, at whatever level, was what mattered most. Many recent studies show similar results.

Surprisingly, cardiorespiratory fitness level didn't matter at all for those who were not active. That is, being aerobically fit provided no protection from coronary heart disease mortality in men who were sedentary. To understand how this could be the case, it is necessary to realize that cardiorespiratory fitness is dependent not just on being aerobically active but also on natural endowment. Some people are born with the genetic makeup for a strong cardiorespiratory system, while others are not, and no amount—or lack—of exercise can entirely override that genetic endowment. Thus, if fitness is measured by cardiorespiratory criteria, it's possible to be fit *and* sedentary. However, what the Copenhagen results show is that a high cardiorespiratory fitness level, as measured by stress tests, is not as good an indicator of longevity as physical activity. So being cardiorespiratorily fit may give you a false sense of security—especially if that fitness comes from natural endowment, rather than from being active.

I'm not saying that the traditional notion of cardiorespiratory fitness, and the means by which it is frequently measured, are without merit. To the contrary, I'm all for cardiorespiratory fitness. It, too, has significant implications for health and longevity, especially *if* it is linked with physical activity. For example, even though it didn't give any of the sedentary men an edge in longevity, it did help the physically active men. Active men who were in the top fifth of the fitness levels had about half the mortality rate of active men who were in the bottom fifth. Several other studies published within the past ten to fifteen years also have shown an inverse relationship between cardiorespiratory fitness level and death rate. In these studies, high fitness levels usually corresponded with high levels of physical activity, suggesting that physical activity itself was important, too. I'm also heartily in favor of muscular fitness, as defined in terms of strength, speed, and power levels, but both cardiorespiratory and muscular fitness have a strong genetic component to them, which you can't do anything about. So even if you work at improving these kinds of fitness, there are real limits to how much improvement you can bring about, limits that can make you feel like a failure and, therefore, abandon all effort.

That's what usually happens when people go on fitness binges. Discouraged by their inability to achieve the aerobic- or strength-training goals they have set for themselves—goals often inspired by their young, athletic fitness instructors—they quit their exercise regimens and lapse once again into inactivity. Thus, they never achieve metabolic fitness, which is almost entirely within their control, easier to achieve, and a better indicator of good health and longevity to boot! It is metabolic fitness that does the most to help minimize the risk of diseases such as atherosclerosis and type 2 diabetes.

Metabolic fitness and the health benefits that come with it are more about being *active* than about being *fit*. You don't have to be a lean machine with the heart and muscles of an athlete to be insulin sensitive, and have normal blood pressure and a great blood-fat profile.

The No-Sweat Way to Metabolic Fitness

In the late 1980s Japanese researchers did an interesting study of the value of metabolic, as opposed to cardiorespiratory, fitness. Though insulin sensitivity was commonly believed to be linked to aerobic capacity, they wanted to see if it was possible to achieve improvements in the former without effecting any change in the latter. Six men, between the ages of eighteen and twenty-two, participated in a very low-intensity exercise program for one year. They jogged two and one-half miles in about 35 minutes, four times per week (for a total of 140 minutes a week, which coincidentally conforms to my recommendation). Since they were exercising at a very low level of intensity—0.55 of maximum heart rate, which is *under* the lowest end of the target heartbeat range—their cardiorespiratory capacity did not improve. Nor did they lose any weight.

By traditional standards this exercise program was a failure, *but not by the standards of metabolic fitness.* After just one month on the program the men's insulin sensitivity improved. By the end of their no-sweat year of exercise, their insulin sensitivity had improved by more than 50 percent; that is, they needed less than half the insulin formerly required to process a given amount of glucose.

It takes less than a year, or even a month, to see exercise-induced enhancement of metabolic fitness. During the past 10 years a number of research groups have demonstrated that insulin sensitivity can be improved substantially within just one week after starting an exercise program—without weight loss and in the absence of improvements in cardiovascular fitness. Muscle activity alone appears to be the key.

As the concept of metabolic, rather than cardiorespiratory, fitness has begun to take hold in the scientific field, there have been more and more studies that report similar findings. Dr. Jean-Pierre Després and his colleagues at Laval University in Quebec have published numerous papers on the benefits conferred by exercise, regardless of whether weight is lost or cardiorespiratory capacity is improved. The scenario for each of their studies was the same. Obese women, usually weighing two hundred pounds or more, were placed on a moderate-intensity exercise program for a period of several months to a year or more. Cardiorespiratory capacity was very little improved, and weight loss was typically less than ten pounds, half or more of it body fat, with all the women still remaining at BMIs well over 30 (meaning they were still obese by U.S. government BMI standards). However, CAT scans show that much of the body fat lost was visceral fat, the kind that is detrimental to health, and, given the relatively small amounts of visceral fat on the body, the amounts lost were actually fairly significant. The improvement in metabolic fitness parameters was quite impressive.

In one such study, women who weighed an average of 215 pounds dropped an average of 5 pounds after six months of light exercise four to five times per week—not much to brag about by conventional standards. However, their triglycerides decreased by 23 percent, and their ratio of HDL cholesterol to LDL cholesterol improved by 14 percent. Moreover, out of the modest five-pound weight loss, three of those pounds were fat, most of it the bad kind.

So, if your goal is to live longer and healthier, rather than thinner, the no-sweat metabolic fitness program is for you.

Before You Start...

All exercise programs begin—or should begin—with a warning about potential risks, even though the risks associated with exercise are far less common and serious than the risks associated with not doing any exercise. However, there are risks, and you need to know what they are in order to make them even more minimal. The first set of dangers consists of possible injuries to your bones, joints, and muscles, including but not limited to some possible soreness when you begin using muscles in ways in which you haven't used them for years. By following a few basic guidelines provided later in the chapter, you can avoid or reduce the possibility of this kind of problem.

The much more serious kind of risk consists of heart attack or sudden death during physical activity. Everyone has heard the horror stories about the sudden death of various high-profile athletes who died on the running track or the basketball court or whatever. Jim Fixx, the celebrated author of *The Complete Book of Running* died while running. Basketball stars Reggie Lewis, Pete Maravich, and Hank Gathers all died while playing basketball. Flo Hyman, U.S. women's Olympics volleyball team star, died during a competition. Indeed such stories are often cited by those who are trying to convince you—or more likely themselves—that exercise is just too dangerous.

However, the risk of sudden death during exercise, while real, is also fairly rare. Current data indicate that each year in the United States fewer than 1 out of 15,000 adults might be expected to die during vigorous exercise. The fact is, the vast majority of heart attacks that occur each year in the United States take place during non-exercise-related activities, such as eating, sleeping, and watching TV. If you do vigorous exercise twenty minutes a day, the slightly increased risk of heart attack during that period is greatly outweighed by the reduction in risk during the other twenty-three hours and forty minutes of the day.

Each of the sudden-death examples cited above had pre-existing cardiac problems that were not created by any sport or exercise. The best way to make sure that you don't fall into the same category is to get a medical checkup before embarking on a new exercise program. *All* women over the age of fifty, and all men over the age of forty, should consult their physicians before increasing their activity level. Regardless of age, anyone considering an exercise program who has experienced chest pains or dizziness or has two or more risk factors for heart disease, such as smoking, high cholesterol, high blood pressure, or a sedentary lifestyle, should consult a doctor. During your checkup your doctor will decide whether or not you should have a stress test. Actually you might want to have a stress test even if you decide to remain sedentary. An eminent physician and exercise physiologist from Sweden, Dr. Per-Olof Astrand, once advised that anyone who had elected a sedentary lifestyle should get a stress test to determine whether he could afford *not* to exercise.

To maximize the benefits of being active, while minimizing the risks, just follow one simple rule: Exercise in moderation. Below, I will explain how to gauge the intensity of your exercise so that you can keep it in the moderate range—or increase it if you choose.

Beyond the Two-Minute Walk

To obtain substantial benefits from your physical activity, you are eventually going to have to get to the twenty-minute-a-day level; if you're really out of shape and have been sedentary for a long time, you should get to that level gradually. During the first week you might decide to do only a few two-minute walks per day. Over the weeks to come, keep upping that amount, until within a month or two you are complying with the twenty-minutes-a-day recommendation. Of course, you can do other activities if you choose. I recommend walking just because it is so convenient, so easy to incorporate into your day, and requires no more of an investment than a pair of comfortable walking shoes.

Don't think that once you get to the goal of 20 minutes per day, you must get in at least 20 minutes every day, and that the 20 minutes must be all in one session. Missing a day or two per week is nothing to worry about; in fact, "rest" days are important so that you don't get run-down. Week-to-week averages of physical activity time are the best measure; just shoot for an average of about 140 minutes per week. Furthermore, as research over the past 10 years has proved, including some that I did recently at the University of Virginia, accumulating shorter bouts of 5-to-10 minutes throughout the day is just as effective as doing the exercise all at one time. In other words, two or three 10-minute walks are just as effective as one 20-to-30-minute walk.

Other ideas for becoming more active are detailed on the next few pages.

Turn Sedentary Activities into Active Ones

For example, instead of making a lunch date with a friend, make an exercise date or a walk date. Taking a walk through the park, or down the block, or to the mall, provides a great chance to catch up with each other and also do yourselves some good.

Another typically sedentary activity that can be converted to an active one is talking on the phone. If you have a cordless phone, you can walk while you're talking. I'm serious. The fittest "walking talker" I know is my wife. She averages at least one hour per day on the phone—in motion. Conservatively, she logs a couple of hundred miles per year on the phone. I call them frequent-dialer miles. They're not around a track, and they don't cause her to break into a sweat, but she goes around the house, up and down the stairs, out into the yard and back in again, logging her unconventional but entirely worthwhile miles. And she is as fit—metabolically and cardiovascularly—as just about any woman her age (and a good many younger ones too). If you don't have a cordless phone, get one, and consider it "exercise equipment." Or get a stationary bike or a treadmill, and log your miles on them while talking on the phone.

You can even make TV watching an aerobic activity. Use the commercial breaks—usually about 2 minutes long—for your 2-minute walks. You could reach your 140-minutes-per-week goal in the space of just 70 commercial breaks—out of the roughly 150 that the average adult sits through each week. (This is based on an average rate of 5 commercial breaks per hour, and the fact that the average U.S. adult watches about 30 hours of TV each week.) Alternately, you could watch TV while using the treadmill or exercise bike. Pick one show per day as your "fitness" show and use that time to exercise. You can also listen to music while on one of these stationary exercisers, or read, or (as noted above) talk on the phone.

Learn to take "longcuts" instead of shortcuts, to take the path of most resistance rather than the path of least resistance. Climb stairs instead of waiting for the elevator. Park your car at the farthest rather than the closest distance in the parking lot. Go out for coffee yourself instead of sending your secretary. Walk the dog yourself instead of getting the children to do it.

Engage in More Recreational Sports and Games

Even sports that were formerly considered to be useless under the old aerobic standards for fitness we now understand to be very much worth doing. Golf, for example, used to be considered not intense enough to promote health because it didn't raise the heart rate high enough, but with the new research demonstrating the health benefits of physical activity at any intensity, it is looking good. As proof, Finnish researchers reported in a 2000 issue of the *American Journal of Medicine* that playing golf two to three times per week (walking the course!) improved cardiovascular endurance, reduced waist circumference, and elevated blood levels of HDL cholesterol (the good kind) in middle-aged men. If you play eighteen holes of golf without riding a cart, just the walking alone can add up to several miles of walking—and that's if you hit straight and stay on the fairway. If you're like me, and don't, then eighteen holes of golf can turn into a veritable marathon. Another advantage of golf is that it can be played well into your senior years. My father is an avid golfer, who has been playing regularly for his whole life, walking the course every time and carrying his own clubs. Why has he continued to walk the course instead of riding, unlike most of his contemporaries? His answer has always been "I like the exercise. Golf wouldn't be the same otherwise." He has probably logged at least ten thousand miles of walking while playing golf. Only recently, at age seventy-five, did he decide to make things easier for himself by using a cart to pull his clubs. Not surprisingly he's as fit as most men twenty years younger. Don't be put off by golf's formerly elitist image. There are now thousands of public golf courses all over the country.

But *any* sport will do. There are sixty-eight different sports activities that can qualify you and your family members (ages six and older) for something called the Presidential Sports Award. Generally speaking, it takes about fifty hours of activity in a given sport within a four-month period of time to qualify—about 25 minutes a day, in other words—and the sports range from aerobic dancing to wrestling, cheerleading to figure skating, tai chi to karate, and they include team as well as individual activities. Successful completion entitles you to a number of goodies, including a certificate from the President. While I realize this may have little appeal to most grown-ups, it's a great way to motivate children to become more active, which may help you to become more active, too, if you use such activities as an opportunity for a bit of family togetherness. For more information, write to Presidential Sports Award, Amateur Athletic Union, Walt Disney World Resort, P.O. Box 10000, Lake Buena Vista, FL 32830-1000, call 407-934-7200, or visit their website at www.*pueblo.gsa.gov/cic_text/health/win-win/presawrd.htm.*

Gradually Incorporate Aerobic Activities into Your Life

The more traditional types of exercise, particularly aerobic, are definitely worth doing. Although the Exercise Lite approach is great for getting the truly sedentary up off their couches, even if just above idling speed, the same research that established that physical activity at any level is good also makes it perfectly clear that more exercise—mostly in terms of duration, but also at a slightly higher intensity—is better. However, this is true only up to a certain point. The law of diminishing returns applies to exercise. What this basically means is that doing twenty minutes per day of physical activity is probably not as beneficial as doing forty, but forty minutes is not twice as good as twenty. The return on your investment does not increase in a straight-line manner.

The person who will enjoy the greatest benefits of all is the one who goes *from nothing to something*—from zero minutes of exercise per day to an average of twenty minutes per day. After that the benefits keep increasing with duration and/or intensity, but never as dramatically as with that first change. This is illustrated by the results of a relatively recent study of the effects of walking on risk of type 2 diabetes among 70,102 women ages thirty to fifty-five. Women who walked an average of between 18 and 33 minutes per day reduced their risk of type 2 diabetes by 27 percent (compared to women who reported essentially no regular physical activity). Women who walked an average of more than 86 minutes per day (that is, nearly an hour and a half per day, or more) reduced their risk of type 2 diabetes by 42 percent. The approximately 50 percent greater reduction in risk required more than three times as much walking to achieve it. Other studies published recently show similar findings for walking and reduced risk of coronary heart disease and stroke.

If you do want additional benefits, walking at a brisk pace, running, swimming, bicycling, or working out on one of the many different kinds of stationary aerobic machines now so popular in fitness clubs, are all excellent activities. For the sake of variety, as well as to minimize any stress on joints or muscles, you might want to switch off among these activities.

No Pain, Lots of Gain: Regulating Intensity

With respect to the more traditional types of exercise—the ones that I just recommended you might want to do more of—the question of intensity always arises. How hard to exercise? In the 1980s Jane Fonda told us to "go for the burn," and for as long as I can remember, I've been hearing the phrase "no pain, no gain," most particularly as it pertains to exercise, but going for the burn in the eighties seems to have done little more than produce a lot of exercise burnouts in the nineties and beyond. Exercise can, and should, be painless. That doesn't mean that it can't be a lot more intense than the moderate, no-sweat kind of exercise I've been talking about for metabolic fitness. But even to achieve endurance and aerobic fitness, it's not necessary to do one of those gut-busting workouts we've all been taught were the only ones worth doing.

I did a study of my own some years ago, as part of my ongoing research effort to find out how much energy you need to put into exercise to get significant benefits. With a grant from the American Heart

Association, I set out to study the impact of exercise intensity on blood pressure, aerobic fitness, body fat, and certain aspects of metabolic fitness (although the concept of metabolic fitness was still in the developmental stages at that time). Sixteen college students who had volunteered for the study were assigned at random to one of two exercise groups, one that would work out at an average of 65 percent of maximum heart rate, the other at an average of 90 percent. All participants exercised just three days a week for four and one-half months, the lower-intensity group for 50 minutes per session (for a total of 150 minutes a week), the higher-intensity group for 25 minutes per session (for a total of 75 minutes per week), so that both groups would burn about the same number of calories.

The striking difference between the two groups was the effort they had to put into achieving their assigned heartbeat range. The higher-intensity group sweated buckets, and could not concentrate on anything but cranking the pedals on their stationary bikes and counting down the minutes until they were finished. They were working so hard, they knew they were really achieving something. By contrast, the lower-intensity group never broke a sweat. Most studied or read newspapers or magazines during their workouts, and barely felt that they were doing real exercise. And no wonder: Their 65 percent of maximum heart rate is *below* the average level (70 percent) that walkers reached when they were told to choose a walking pace that was natural to them, according to a study conducted by researchers at the University of South Carolina.

Like my subjects, I expected that the effort they put into exercise would be reflected in the benefits they got out of it, and hence anticipated little change in any of the fitness indicators for the lower-intensity group. However, I was wrong. For example, both groups improved their average aerobic fitness levels, as measured by exercise stress tests, by the same amount, about 17 to 20 percent, and the people in both groups lost an average of 3 pounds of body fat apiece.

All of the young men showed improvement in at least some indicator of metabolic fitness: reduced blood pressure, decreased LDL cholesterol, or increased HDL cholesterol, with improvements typically being in the range of 5 to 15 percent—and no connection appearing between amount of improvement and level of exercise intensity. *In fact, there was no connection between level of intensity and changes in any of the indicators I was measuring, which included blood pressure, blood fats, aerobic capacity, and amount of body fat.* What I did notice, however—and this is in line with the "diminishing returns" principle noted above—was that those who improved the most were those whose indicators were the worst to begin with. Thus, the men with the highest pre-exercise LDL cholesterol levels were the ones who reduced them the most; and the men with the lowest HDL cholesterol levels achieved the biggest increases, without regard to intensity of exercise.

Another interesting thing I noted was that these improvements were brought about in the higher-intensity group in even less time per week—75 minutes—than the 140 I'm recommending. Though I think most people beyond college age aren't going to want to do that kind of exercise—and certainly anybody who does should be absolutely sure to get a stress test beforehand—if you do opt for high-intensity exercise, it allows you to make efficient use of your time. The general moral is: Do what suits you. Either exercise at lower intensity for longer periods or get it over with as fast as possible by doing a much harder workout (pending your doctor's approval).

There are a number of ways of calculating intensity of exercise, including the heart-rate-per-minute criterion that we've been discussing, and something called the Rating of Perceived Exertion (RPE) scale, which was developed by Swedish researcher Gunnar Borg (and is also called the Borg scale). The Borg scale rates exertion from 0 to 10 as indicated below:

Score	Perceived Exertion
0	Nothing at all (at rest)
0.5	Very, very weak
1	Very weak
2	Weak
3	Moderate
4	Somewhat strong
5	Strong
6	
7	Very strong
8	
9	
10	Very, very strong (maximal, exhausting)

A few years after the study on college-age men, I conducted another one at the City of Hope Medical Center in Duarte, California, which showed how these scores tend to correspond to heart rates. This time my colleagues and I were studying seventeen men and women between the ages of sixty-five and seventy-five. We assessed cardiorespiratory fitness improvements in two different, randomly assigned groups—a lower-intensity group, who walked for thirty minutes at 65 percent of maximum heart rate; and a higher-intensity group, who walked at close to 90 percent. Perception matched up nicely with actuality. Subjects in the lower-intensity group rated their exertion between a 1 and a 3 on the Borg scale, those in the higher-intensity group were typically closer to a 6 or a 7.

Though some of the people in the lower-intensity group were upset that they weren't doing more vigorous exercise—after all, they had volunteered for the study because they thought they were going to get fit—they were mollified when they saw the results. After eight weeks of four-times-a-week walking sessions, everyone had achieved improvements in cardiorespiratory fitness, and the lower-intensity group had done just as well as the higher-intensity group. Even though their level of exertion hadn't felt like exercise to them, it was, but it was the new-wave kind— no pain, lots of gain.

Many studies have shown similar results. The ACSM itself now says that training at lower intensities has been shown to lower blood pressure as much as (or even more than) training at higher intensities. Suffice it to say that if you are exercising at an intensity that makes it hard for you to have a conversation, you are exercising harder than you need to.

Warming Up, Cooling Down, and Stretching

In order to minimize your risk of injury and harm, especially if you're moving beyond the moderate-intensity level of exercise, you'll want to do a warm-up and a cool-down, as well as some stretching exercises. Though many people, including fitness instructors, confuse stretching with warming up, the best way of warming up is simply to start doing your exercise, but at a very low level of intensity, for several minutes. Increase to the desired intensity at a gradual pace. If you exercise in the morning, just after getting up, it may take longer to work out the kinks, in which case you should take longer to warm up.

Stretching should be done either after your exercise session is over or, better yet, after a few minutes of warming up. It's best not to *begin* your exercise session by stretching, because until your muscles and tendons are warm, they'll be less pliable and flexible, therefore more prone to tearing. Some other general rules about stretching are: Never bounce when you stretch; stretch just to the point of slight-to-moderate resistance, not to the point of pain; and once you've gotten to the slight-to-moderate resistance level, hold the stretch for between ten and thirty seconds. For more information about stretching I recommend buying a good how-to book, one with lots of pictures depicting a variety of stretching positions. Bob Anderson's classics—*Stretching: 20th Anniversary, Revised Edition*, and *Stretching at Your Computer or Desk*—are terrific. There are many other good books on the subject as well.

Cooling down is particularly important after vigorous exercise, because it allows your heart and circulatory system to slow down gradually. Sudden stops can result in faintness, especially if you stand motionless, allowing the blood to pool in the lower part of your body. So keep your muscles working at a low level of intensity for a few minutes after you've completed the target-heart-range portion of your session. If you're doing only light-to-moderate exercise, however, the cool-down is not essential.

A typical 30- to 40-minute exercise session, complete with warm-up, stretch, and cool-down would go something like this: Warm up for 3 to 5 minutes, do some easy stretching for 5 minutes, do the activity itself for 20 to 25 minutes, and cool down for a few minutes at the end. Do three or four of these sessions a week, which still keeps you within the 140 minutes or so that I said would be effective, and you're finished. Anything more is great. Or you may choose to break up the 30-to-40-minute sessions into several shorter bouts of 5-to-10 minutes that might fit more easily into your busy daily routine. Both alternatives work just the same.

If you find that you can fit something else into the week's activities, strength training would be a particularly valuable addition. Strength training, also known as weight lifting or resistance training, is not just for bodybuilders or the superfit. Because we start to lose muscle mass as we age, particularly after our thirties, it can be particularly valuable for people middle-aged and older. For them it can help both to prevent further muscle shrinkage and loss and to restore muscle that has been neglected from years of disuse. Strong muscles are important for balance, for injury prevention, and certainly for enjoying and getting the most out of daily life. Recent studies show that strength training can also increase insulin sensitivity and helps maintain and/or enhance bone density.

The good news is that strength training can bring about significant improvements at any age, even in the elderly, for loss of muscle mass is due not just to the natural aging process, but also to disuse. *Use it or lose it* is absolutely accurate when it comes to muscle mass (and probably to bone density too). You can find strength-training courses at many parks and recreation departments, at Y's, at community colleges, and at gyms and health clubs. Or you can use an illustrated book on the subject to get you started. A very user-friendly strength-training starter program can be found in one of my other books, *The Spark: The Revolutionary New Plan to Get Fit and Lose Weight 10 Minutes at a Time* (Fireside, 2002). This plan is designed for beginners and is especially suited for those who don't have big chunks of time during the day for exercise.

Making Sure You Succeed

To maintain a program of regular physical activity, give yourself all the help you can. In my opinion, the most helpful thing you could do would be to form a support group of like-minded friends and family members who share your commitment to being more active. I run regularly with several of my colleagues at the University of Virginia. Schedules change from day to day, so we can never be sure when we might go. But without question, by noon one of us will call someone in the group and ask, "What time are we going?" Not "*Are* we running?" but "*When?*" It makes it difficult to say no, even in the face of inertia or overwork. If those in your support group make time for you, you make time for them.

Exercise can be a family activity, too, thus keeping the parents active and giving them a chance to set good examples for their children. My wife and I run together. With young children this poses a problem of childcare. We solved that by taking them to the track with us. While we run around the track, the kids play on the infield grass or in the sandboxes. (Note: Long jump pits make great sandboxes.) It works out fine, and the lesson sinks in, as I saw with our oldest boy. For years he accompanied us to the track without ever showing any inclination to join us, and without our ever pressing him to. Then one day, out of the blue, when he was twelve years old, he announced that he wanted to do a ten-kilometer run. He had just suddenly gotten the urge. Although I discouraged him from trying, since he had had no training, he did it. The results weren't terrific that first time, but he decided to keep at it. Six years later, after a lot of training, he was able to run a 4:15 mile, and he placed third in the California State High School Cross-Country Championship.

It's Never Too Late to Start

Just as it's never too early, it's never too late to start. The benefits of physical activity are always available to us, at any age. Several studies published within the past ten years—-a couple from ongoing studies described earlier in the book—make this clear.

Dr. Steven Blair has been studying the effects of physical fitness on mortality rates since 1970 at the Cooper Institute in Dallas, with results that consistently show the value of exercise (see Chapter 4). In one particularly relevant report from this ongoing study, published in the April 12, 1995, issue of the *Journal of the American Medical Association*, Dr. Blair and his colleagues describe the results of a study they did on 9,777 men, each of whom was given two stress tests sometime between 1970 and 1989, and then followed for an average of five years after their second test. The purpose of this follow-up period was to assess any changes in mortality rates due to changes in fitness levels. The mortality results showed that those who had been deemed "unfit" on the basis of the first stress test, who had then increased their physical activity and thereby become "fit" at the time of the second stress test, experienced a 44 percent reduction in premature death rates. Significantly, improved longevity had nothing to do with weight loss. Men who had a BMI above 27 at the first examination but below 27 at the second had a slightly higher (though not statistically significant) death rate.

Dr. Blair's findings are confirmed by those of Dr. Ralph Paffenbarger, in a follow-up on the men of the Harvard Alumni study. As reported in the February 25, 1993, *New England Journal of Medicine*, Paffenbarger and his research team found that men who were relatively sedentary when the study began, in the early 1960s, but who had increased their physical activity level by taking up moderate sports by the time the follow-up began in 1977, experienced a 23 percent lower mortality rate in the years 1977-85, compared with men who were sedentary to begin with and remained so. Most importantly, the reduction in mortality rate was observed in men of all ages, from their forties through their eighties. It's never too late to become active, or to get the benefits of being active.

Two additional studies, one from Great Britain and one from Norway, and both published in 1998, bear out the findings from the U.S. studies. The British researchers found that "taking up light or moderate physical activity reduces mortality and heart attacks in older men with and without diagnosed cardiovascular disease." The Norwegian researchers emphasized that "even small improvements in physical fitness are associated with a significantly lowered risk of death."

If, despite all the evidence, you remain adamantly antiexercise, even at the two-minute walk level, there is still a lot you can do to improve your health. The second component of the Twenty/Twenty Program is the set of nutritional recommendations in the following chapter. Since those who stand to benefit most from the program are those who are at greatest risk, any improvement at all, in activity level or eating habits, is important. In the Twenty/Twenty Program, just getting close counts, as it does in horseshoes (which, by the way, is one of the physical activities that can win you a Presidential Sports Award).

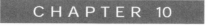

CHAPTER 10

Nutrition for Metabolic Fitness

The major cause of death in the United States is food poisoning. It is not the kind of food poisoning that you usually think about. Our food poisoning comes from the normal foods in our diet.

—Nathan Pritikin, *The Humanist*, 1984

Before you read any farther, stop. Put down the book again. Now go eat something, as long as it's something relatively high in complex carbohydrates and fiber and with relatively little fat or sugar. Any of the following will do just fine: most any fruit; a handful of any raw vegetables, such as carrots, red or green peppers, or celery; a half-cup of three-bean salad (without oil); or some wholesome grain product, such as a slice of whole wheat bread, a bagel, or a low-fat bran muffin. You could even have a small bowl of air-popped popcorn.

Believe it or not, this is a key step in following the nutritional part of the Twenty/Twenty Program, because the emphasis in this program is not just on *eating less* fat, but also on *eating more*—healthier alternatives such as more fruit, more vegetables, more grains, and more legumes (which are another kind of vegetable, in the form of dried beans, lentils, or peas). While it's true that many of our nutritional problems—the food "poisoning" to which Nathan Pritikin was referring—are caused by eating too much fat, they are also related to eating too few complex carbohydrates. This deprives our bodies of all the good stuff that comes with them, such as fiber, antioxidant vitamins, and literally thousands of cancer-fighting compounds called phytochemicals (literally, "plant chemicals," which you can't get in a pill).

Improving insulin sensitivity—the core of metabolic fitness—is one of the major goals of this program. Although we do not completely understand how various foods affect the body's responsiveness to insulin, this much can be said with assurance: Diets high in fat, especially saturated fat, tend to impair insulin sensitivity, and diets high in complex carbohydrate and fiber tend to have the opposite effect. The different kinds of fat (saturated and unsaturated) and the different kinds of carbohydrates (simple and complex) are explained in the next section.

Carbohydrates and Fats: Some Definitions

Carbohydrates—Simple and Complex

When I say to eat more carbohydrates, I'm referring mainly to the complex carbohydrates. The simple carbohydrates are sugars such as are found in table sugar and honey (and also in fruit). Complex carbohydrates are long "chains" (polymers) of hundreds of thousands, or even millions, of simple sugars, and they are found in two forms in our foods: *starch* and *fiber*. Starches are abundant in grains—grains being the basic material of cereal, bread, pasta, and rice—and in legumes. Fiber makes up much of the bulk of most of our fruits and vegetables, and is also abundant in grains and legumes. We need carbohydrates for energy. They fuel the brain and the nervous system, and they are your muscles' preferred fuel during exercise, especially vigorous exercise.

Saturated Fats

Though all dietary fats have the same number of calories (9 per gram), not all fats are created equal in other respects. Some fats, in limited quantities, are good for you and essential to your health. Besides its value as a concentrated source of energy, fat is necessary for hormone function, vitamin absorption, and immune system activities. Saturated fat, for the most part, is the bad kind, the kind most particularly implicated in increased cholesterol levels and decreased sensitivity to insulin (insulin resistance).

Saturated fats are found mainly in animal products, and also in palm, palm kernel, and coconut oils. Foods with large amounts of saturated fat include red meat, liver, whole milk and whole-milk products (like cheese and yogurt), chocolate, eggs, cream, butter, cocoa butter, and the above-mentioned oils. Hamburger meat and whole milk rank as the two greatest contributors of saturated fat to the American diet. Just by making the switch from whole milk to skim milk (2 cups per day), and from a ground beef with 20 to 25 percent fat to one with under 10 percent fat (one three-ounce serving per day), the average American could reduce his or her fat intake from about 35 percent to 27 percent of total calories. Such a reduction in fat consumption has been reported to prevent the build-up of fatty deposits on arterial walls, and also reduce blood pressure—even in the absence of weight loss, as demonstrated in the Cholesterol Lowering Atherosclerosis Study and the Dietary Approaches to Stop Hypertension clinical trial, mentioned in Chapter 3.

Unsaturated Fats

These fats, the *good* fats (as long as complex carbohydrates still dominate the diet), are found mainly in fish, nuts, olives, avocados, and vegetable oils, and can be either monounsaturated or poly-unsaturated. While there has been considerable back-and-forthing about which kind is better for you, monounsaturated seems to be winning for now, but both kinds of fat appear to be helpful in lowering cholesterol levels. Oils high in monounsaturated fat include olive, almond, canola, and peanut.

Olive oil, of course, has been hogging all the attention in recent years, because of its hypothesized link to the greater longevity of people who live in countries along the northern coast of the Mediterranean—in Greece, and in the south of Italy, France, and Spain. The Mediterranean diet, as the food eaten by these people is now referred to, is indeed very high in monounsaturated fat, principally from olive oil. While this is a diet relatively high in fat—30 to 40 percent of daily intake, just like ours—the people who eat it have heart disease rates much lower than ours. As a result, many researchers are now looking to olive oil as a possible key to longevity. However, my own speculation is that the most important difference between our diet and the Mediterranean diet is not the olive oil consumption, but the consumption of a number of other foods. The Mediterranean diet typically consists of about twice as much fruit and seafood as ours, two-thirds more vegetables, one-fifth more grains and beans, and only half as much meat.

Oils high in polyunsaturated fats include corn, cottonseed, safflower, sesame, soybean, sunflower, and walnut. Fish oils, mainly those from cold-water fish such as salmon, mackerel, herring, sardines, tuna, anchovies, swordfish, trout, halibut, and bluefish, are also high in polyunsaturated fats, including the much-touted *omega-3 fatty acids*, as are oysters, shrimp, and lobster. These polyunsaturated fatty acids have been reported to lower the risk of heart attacks by making the blood less likely to clot, and perhaps by reducing cholesterol levels and having a modest blood-pressure-lowering effect as well. The best way to get your omega-3 fatty acids is by eating fish, and not by use of supplements.

One exception to the "unsaturated fat is good fat" rule is the kind of fat typically contained in margarine: hydrogenated oil. You'll find by reading the package that most sticks or tubs of margarine contain partially-hydrogenated vegetable oil. Hydrogenation is a process that causes oil to harden at room temperature, which makes it closer in chemical makeup to a saturated fat than to an unsaturated fat, even though it is made from vegetable oil. Hydrogenated vegetable oils (also called "trans fats" or "trans fatty acids") are now widely used in many products, especially candy, baked goods, and baking mixes, because they lengthen shelf life and improve the texture of foods. However, we may be paying a price for those advantages—hydrogenated oils have been shown to reduce the levels of HDL cholesterol and raise the levels of LDL cholesterol in our blood. Some brands of margarine now are made without hydrogenated fat; these tub margarines will have "zero trans fats" indicated on the container. If you use a lot of processed, packaged foods, however, it will be difficult to avoid them entirely.

Whether a fat is a "good fat" or a "bad fat," whether it lowers cholesterol or raises it, the best approach to fat, if you consume the average American diet, is to eat less of it. Whatever cholesterol reduction you could achieve by eating more olive oil, for example, would be extremely modest in comparison with the improvements you could effect by eating more complex carbohydrates instead.

Starting the Nutrition Component of the Twenty/Twenty Program: The High-Carbohydrate Way to Health

"Substantial public health and clinical benefits could be achieved simply by increasing the public's consumption of fruits and vegetables," said Dr. Gladys Block, professor of public health, U.C. Berkeley, in a statement that reflects a growing consensus about the poor state of the American diet—and what could be done to improve it. What could be simpler? Yet few Americans consume the U.S. dietary recommendations regarding fruits and vegetables, which call for two to four servings of fruit, and three to five servings of vegetables per day. (See the section on the "Food Guide Pyramid" below.) Approximately one person in three meets the minimum recommendation for vegetables alone; only one in five meets the minimum recommendation for fruit. Children ages 2 to 18 average only 2.6 servings of vegetables and 1.6 servings of fruit per day. As a result of our poor vegetable and fruit consumption, we consume an average of less than 15 grams of fiber per day, which falls well short of the 20 to 35 grams recommended by the National Cancer Institute. This is why the 20 percent fat goal of my Twenty/Twenty Program has as much to do with getting you to eat more as it does with getting you to eat less.

Even if you don't cut one single gram of fat from your diet, just try this for starters: Eat at least one or two extra helpings of fruit, and one or two extra servings of vegetables (not including French fries or anything else fried) per day, especially if you currently fall short of the daily recommended minimums. Spread them out over the day; treat them as snacks. You'll be healthier for it. Besides the fact that you'll be ingesting more food that is good for you, you'll be doing it in a healthier way: *nibbling*. Eating small snacks throughout the day, as opposed to eating just at regular mealtimes, can lower your cholesterol level (especially LDL) and improve insulin sensitivity, even if you don't cut fat or total calories.

More than one hundred studies published in the past few decades have shown that people who eat a lot of fruits and vegetables have only about one-half the risk of cancer compared with people who don't—

namely, the majority of Americans. Furthermore, because of the high-fiber content of fruits and vegetables, eating just two to three servings from these food groups (in addition to, not in place of, the other foods you eat) can also provide you with enough fiber to greatly reduce your risk of heart disease, as the following studies suggest.

In 1972 researchers at the University of California, San Diego (UCSD) Medical School asked 859 men and women between the ages of fifty and seventy-nine to fill out questionnaires asking them about their food habits. The researchers then tracked their subjects through 1985, assessing the influence of dietary fiber in coronary heart disease mortality. What they found was that the people who consumed 16 grams or more of fiber per day had a mortality rate from heart disease that was only about *one-third* that of their counterparts, who ate less than 16 grams. In fact, each additional 6 grams of dietary fiber per day was associated with a 25 percent reduction in coronary heart disease rates.

More recently, Nurses' Health Study researchers reported in the June 2, 1999, issue of the *Journal of the American Medical Association* that each 5-gram per day increase in cereal fiber consumption corresponded to a 37 percent lower risk of coronary heart disease. Just one cup of bran flakes, raisin bran, or shredded wheat, for example, contains that much fiber.

These 25-to-37-percent reductions in heart disease risk, by the way, are equal to or greater in magnitude than the reduction that Dr. Paffenbarger and his colleagues observed in Harvard alumni who upped their physical activity level (see Chapter 9). So you see why I say that even if you don't follow both components of the Twenty/Twenty Program, which is how you'll get maximum benefits, you'll still achieve considerable health improvements from following just one—or parts of one.

The UCSD Medical School researchers' findings about the impact of fiber on heart disease are probably explained by a number of short-term studies that have shown significant improvement in blood-fat levels with the addition of fiber to the diet. (Note: These studies are not about fiber supplements, but fiber in the form of *food.*) Just 5 to 6 additional grams of fiber per day have been shown to lower total cholesterol, mainly by lowering the bad kind (LDL) by 10 to 15 mg/dl, which amounts to about 10 percent of the average LDL cholesterol level.

The effect of fiber was independent of all other dietary factors studied by the UCSD Medical School researchers, including total calories, and total fat and cholesterol consumption. Hence my suggestion that even if you don't reduce your fat intake, you might choose to increase your intake of fruits, vegetables, legumes, and fiber-rich grains. That half-cup of three-bean salad I suggested at the start of this chapter can give you close to 6 grams of fiber; so can three slices of most breads, a cup of shredded wheat or raisin bran cereal, a couple cups of strawberries or blueberries, a large orange or grapefruit, two large pears, or three small kiwis.

Besides the good news about cholesterol-lowering effects, many other studies have shown that high-carbohydrate, high-fiber diets improve insulin sensitivity, and reduce blood insulin levels, in a matter of days or weeks. With a critical mass of evidence showing improvements in all these various measures of metabolic fitness, it makes sense that the results add up to a lower incidence of, and mortality from, cancer and heart disease. So you can see why I say, "Eat up."

Eating More Complex Carbohydrates Won't Make You Gain Weight

Every time I make a simple recommendation to eat *more*—as long as it's more fruits, vegetables, and grain products—the inevitable question arises: "Won't I gain weight?" The answer is, "No." First, the human body has a very hard time converting carbohydrates that you eat into fat stored in your fat cells. Carbohydrates tend to get used immediately for energy, not stored, and even when they are stored, they're stored mainly as carbohydrates in your muscle cells, not as fat. Elaborate metabolic experiments have shown that when the body ingests an excess of carbohydrates, even as much as 2,000 calories at a single time, very little of it finds its way into the fat cells. This is the opposite of what happens with fat, which the body stores—in fat cells—with the greatest of ease. Second, carbohydrates tend to have a potent effect on stimulating the metabolism. This "thermic effect" results in additional calories burned. With relatively few exceptions, our bodies just don't seem to be able to gain weight on a high-carbohydrate diet, even if we feed them more calories than they're accustomed to, and even if this "overeating" is extended for a considerable period of time.

There is no shortage of research to demonstrate this fact. One particularly compelling study, published in a 1991 issue of the *American Journal of Clinical Nutrition*, found that it was virtually impossible to gain weight on a high-carbohydrate, low-fat diet. At the University of Illinois at Chicago, eighteen women between the ages of twenty and forty-eight, with BMIs ranging from 18 to 44, consumed a diet consisting of 20 percent fat for a period of twenty weeks, so that researchers could assess its impact on weight and body fat. All meals were prepared for the women by nutritionists in the Nutrition and Metabolism Research Laboratory at the university, so that the percentage of fat in the diet, and the total calories, could be strictly controlled. Since the women's average fat intake before the experiment was 37 percent (which is close to the typical American's), the researchers adjusted the overall quantity of food upward, to make up for the fact that a considerable amount of calorie-rich fat was being removed from the diet. With 1 gram of fat containing 9 calories, and 1 gram of carbohydrate or protein containing 4, it's obvious that a lot more food has to be consumed to keep the level of calories constant when the amount of fat is reduced.

During the course of the twenty weeks, the researchers kept adjusting the food—and calorie—intake upward, to see how much could be consumed on a low-fat diet without resulting in weight gain. But not only was there no weight gain, they couldn't prevent weight *loss*, even though the women ended up consuming an average of 27,000 calories more than their usual intake during a comparable period of time. By the final portion of the twenty weeks, the women were eating an average of 350 more calories per day, but they had lost an average of 4.5 pounds.

The six women who initially weighed the most posted the most impressive results. Despite eating more than 41,000 "extra" calories over the course of the twenty weeks (an average of about 295 calories per day), they, too, lost about 4.5 pounds. Yet, according to the well-known and much-cited principle that 3,500 calories is equivalent to 1 pound of fat, these women should have *gained* 11.7 pounds (41,000 divided by 3,500), not *lost* 4.5. However, not just any calories make you fat; fat calories do that job. On their 20 percent fat diet, these women were consuming about 26 fewer grams of fat per day than they had on their 37 percent fat diet.

I must emphasize that it's not just any kind of high-carbohydrate, low-fat diet that works, as shown by a report in the January 2002 issue of the *American Journal of Clinical Nutrition*. Twenty-seven women and 12 men, all overweight or obese, were assigned to one of three groups that were studied before and after six months of nutrition intervention. The control group consumed their normal diet (about 36 percent fat). The other two groups replaced 25 percent of their daily fat intake with carbohydrates; one group upped only its intake of simple carbohydrates (from 19 percent to 34 percent of total calories) and the other group upped only its intake of complex, fiber-rich carbohydrates (from 21 percent to 33 percent of total calories). All groups were instructed to not consciously reduce their calorie intake. After six months, *only the group that consumed the high-complex-carbohydrate diet lost weight—an average of a little over 9 pounds.* The group that replaced fat with simple carbohydrates did not lose weight despite the fact that the eight women and six men in this group reduced fat intake from 36.5 percent to 20.2 percent of total calories (which was actually slightly more than the reduction in fat intake reported for the group that replaced fat with complex carbohydrates—36.0 percent to 24.6 percent). So "high-fiber" is more important than "low-fat," and this is why I stress the importance of *complex* carbohydrates, typically rich in fiber.

The moral of the story: Don't be the least bit concerned about consuming a few more servings of fruits, vegetables, beans, or grains. The extra calories will not make you gain weight. In reality, though, most people will naturally reduce their fat intake when they consume more fiber-rich foods. Most people, as a result, usually lose a little weight when they focus on consuming more fiber-rich carbohydrates. Regardless of weight, you'll be a lot healthier for the effort. A review of all the popular diets, published in the April 2001 issue of the *Journal of the American Dietetic Association*, found that diet quality was "highest for the high carbohydrate groups and lowest for the low carbohydrate groups." (BMIs were also lowest for men and women consuming high carbohydrate diets and highest for those consuming low carbohydrate diets.)

How to Figure out How Many Grams of Fat Equal 20 Percent

If your fat intake is well above 30 percent, as it is for the majority of Americans, then adding some fruits and vegetables is a good start on improving metabolic fitness—but only a start. Ideally, your fat intake should be close to 20 percent. To do this, you need to have at least a rough idea of your total calorie intake, because the amount of fat intake is a percentage of your daily calorie consumption; and you need to learn how to keep track of your total fat grams—at least initially. If you're like most Americans, you already know a lot about calorie-counting, and probably have a well-thumbed calorie-counter on your bookshelf already. You can keep track of your calories for a few days to get an idea of how many you consume, rely on past records of your average daily food intake, or just use the same estimates of daily calorie intake that most food labels do: 2,000 calories for the average woman, and 2,500 for the average man. If you think you eat either more or fewer calories than these averages, then you can raise or lower your calorie estimate accordingly.

For purposes of showing how to determine how much fat you should be eating in order to get close to 20 percent of the total calorie intake, let's assume the above averages. On a 2,000-calorie-per-day diet, 20 percent works out to 400 calories of fat (2,000 times 0.20). Since 1 gram of fat—any kind of fat—contains 9 calories, 400 calories is equivalent to about 44 grams of fat (400 divided by 9 = 44.4). On a 2,500-calorie-per-day diet, 20 percent works out to about 56 grams of fat. Even if you're off in your counting by 5 or 10 grams or so, it won't make a lot of difference: 54 grams of fat per day instead of 44 on a 2,000-calorie diet, and 67 grams of fat per day on a 2,500-calorie diet, work out to 24 percent fat—still an excellently low level of fat consumption.

Here's what 24 percent will do for you: When researchers at the National Public Health Institute in Helsinki, Finland, put a group of men and women on a 24 percent fat diet, down from their customary 39 percent, after just six weeks the thirty men dropped their average cholesterol from 263 to 201 mg/dl, and the twenty-four women dropped from 239 to 188 mg/dl. These marked decreases are similar in magnitude to those observed on very low fat diets. So, if you keep within a ballpark range of 40 to 50 grams of fat per day out of a 2,000 calorie total, and 55 to 65 grams of fat out of 2,500 calories, you'll be doing great.

Unlike calorie counting, the concept of fat-gram counting may be unfamiliar, even to those of you who have done a lot of dieting, because most diets focus simply on lowering total calories. However, it has become much simpler to keep track of fat intake, thanks to the new food labels, which have been mandatory on all packaged foods since 1994. These labels provide you with useful information about the nutritional and caloric content of various foods, but the single piece of information we're most interested in for present purposes is the fat-gram content. From milk to mayonnaise, cake mix to cookie dough, puff pastry to frozen pizza, creamed corn to canned tuna, every can, box, and jar of food is supposed to bear a label telling you the fat content, by gram, per serving (as well as information about total calorie, protein, carbohydrate, fiber, sugar, cholesterol, and sodium content per serving).

You do need to note the serving size because your definition of a serving may not be the same as the label writer's, but that's an easy matter to deal with. If the label on the water-packed canned tuna says there's 1 gram of fat in a 2-ounce serving and you're eating the whole 6-ounce can for lunch, then you know your fat total is 3 grams. (Obviously, if you add 3 tablespoons of mayonnaise to make tuna salad, you'll have to add another 33 grams of fat, bringing you within range of your recommended total for the day!)

Besides spelling out the number of fat grams, the labels may also use one of the following phrases, each of which means something very specific about fat content:

"Fat-free": less than 1/2 gram of fat per serving.

"Low-fat": 3 grams or less of fat per serving.

"Reduced fat": 25 percent less fat, or one-third fewer calories, than is contained in a comparable food.

"Light" (or "Lite"): 50 percent less fat than in a similar product.

"Lean" and "Extra lean", as they pertain to meat, poultry, or seafood:

"Lean": less than 10 grams of fat, with less than 4 grams of saturated fat and less than 95 milligrams of cholesterol, per 100 gram serving (which is a little less than 3.5 ounces).

"Extra Lean": less than 5 grams of fat, with less than 2 grams of saturated fat and less than 95 milligrams of cholesterol, per 100 gram serving.

Misleading Labels: Weight *versus* Calorie Percentages

Although, in general, food labels are helpful, they can still be tricky to decipher. Perhaps the most confusing of all labels are the ones on products such as milk and meat that say things like "2 percent milk fat" or "90 percent fat-free." Sounds great, doesn't it, if you're trying to get down to a 20 percent fat intake? But it's labels like these that make me continue to focus on counting actual fat grams, because these percentages don't mean what you think they mean. When I recommend a daily fat intake of 20 percent, I mean that the calories from fat should constitute 20 percent of the *total calories* you consume each day. When a milk label says 2 percent fat, it's not talking about a percentage of *calories*, but a percentage of *weight*. So while it's true that fat makes up only 2 percent of the total *weight* of the milk—milk being almost 90 percent water—the *calorie* percentage is quite different. If you happen to have a quart of 2 percent fat milk in your refrigerator, check the label, and you'll see that one serving of milk is something like 120 calories, and the "calories from fat" about 45. The 45 calories of fat constitute 37.5 percent of the *total calories*. Perhaps the reason whole milk (at "3.5 percent fat") and 2 percent fat milk are still so heavily consumed is that people don't understand what they are drinking. Skim milk, which is almost fat-free (under 5 percent of its *calories* are from fat), and 1 percent fat milk (with about 20 percent of its *calories* from fat) are better choices.

A similar confusion prevails in meat labeling. "Lean" ground beef, which can be advertised as "90% lean," or "10% fat," sounds good for someone shooting for a 20 percent fat intake. But meat, like milk, is mainly water (about two-thirds), which has no caloric value, and once again the percentages the package is trumpeting are percentages of *weight*, not *calories*. Thus, "lean" ground beef is really about 50 percent fat if it's calories that are being considered, not weight. Regular ground chuck— "80% lean"—is about 70 percent fat.

The percentage by weight seems to me to be a completely irrelevant piece of information, which is there just to confuse us into buying things we might not otherwise want. Be that as it may, if you keep your focus on *total fat grams per day*, and what percentage they make up of your actual daily calorie total, you can use the food labels successfully.

An additional reason for focusing on fat-gram totals on the labels and ignoring the various pieces of information that pertain to percentages is that food-label "Daily Values" are based on the U.S. recommendation of a fat-percentage target of close to 30 percent—not the 20 to 25 percent that numerous studies indicate is a much healthier level. For example, the 2-percent-milk label tells you that the fat content of a 1-cup serving is 5 grams and that that is 8 percent of the recommended Daily Value, based on a 2,000-calorie diet. However, if you're trying for a 20 percent fat intake, 5 grams is closer to 12 percent than to 8 percent of your daily intake.

One final reason for ignoring the percentages on food labels is that you don't actually need to be interested in what percentage of any given food is made up of fat. You're not trying to assemble a diet made up of foods that all have a fat composition of 20 percent; rather, you're trying to achieve a balance of foods, some high-fat, some low-fat, some no fat, that together add up to a fat total of about 20 percent. The best way of doing this is by counting fat grams.

You will probably be glad that I don't intend for you to do this counting every day for the rest of your life. That would be too tedious, and you would most likely give up almost immediately. If you *can* stand to monitor yourself for a few days, just to get an idea of how much fat (and fiber) you actually eat in a typical day, you'll soon be able to get by with only an occasional glance at a food label.

You may, however, want to get a fat-gram counter, especially if you eat a lot of meals in restaurants or do a lot of cooking from scratch, because if you don't use a lot of packaged, processed foods, you can't look to food labels for the information you need. Bookstores have a number of these on their shelves, many in inexpensive paperback formats. See which one speaks best to your needs, for some focus on fast foods and packaged foods, some give a lot of information on ethnic foods, some will be particularly helpful if you eat often in restaurants, and so forth. Another source of information is the Internet. A number of websites offer a wealth of useful information. One of my favorites is the Tufts Nutrition Navigator at *www.navigator.tufts.edu*; it rates all of the top nutrition websites and has links to all of them. Another great website is the Wheat Foods Council's "Grains Nutrition Information Center" (*www.wheatfoods.org*).

If you don't want to count fat grams at all, then see the Tips section I've included in this chapter for lots of easy-to-follow suggestions on cutting fat from your diet. You may not get all the way down to 20 percent, but you can still achieve some substantial reductions, and with them some very real improvements in health.

Food Guide Pyramid

A Guide to Daily Food Choices

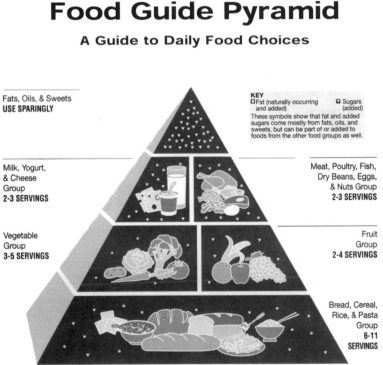

SOURCE: U.S. Department of Agriculture/U.S. Department of Health and Human Services

Use the Food Guide Pyramid to help you eat better every day. . .the Dietary Guidelines way. Start with plenty of Breads, Cereals, Rice, and Pasta; Vegetables; and Fruits. Add two to three servings from the Milk group and two to three servings from the Meat group.

Each of these food groups provides some, but not all, of the nutrients you need. No one food group is more important than another — for good health you need them all. Go easy on fats, oils, and sweets, the foods in the small tip of the Pyramid.

Getting to 20 Percent Fat with the Help of the USDA Food Guide Pyramid

In 1992, the U.S. Department of Agriculture (USDA) released a new set of dietary guidelines in the form of what was called the Food Guide Pyramid. As you can see from the diagram, the Pyramid is divided into six different food groups, with the bottom of the pyramid made up of foods you should be eating the most of; the top, foods you should be eating the least of. At the bottom you see grains, for which the recommended number of servings is between six and eleven. At the top you see fats and sweets, for which there are *no recommended servings*—simply the advice to "use sparingly." You can use the USDA guidelines, in combination with the information I provide about calorie and fat-gram totals per serving of foods within each of the six groups, to help get your fat intake down to something close to 20 percent. It's easier than you think.

Grains: Bread, Cereal, Rice, and Pasta (6-11 servings)

Serving size: 1 slice bread; 1/2 bagel or English muffin; 1 ounce ready-to-eat cereal; 1/2 cup cooked cereal, rice, noodles, or spaghetti; 3 or 4 small, or 2 large, crackers.

Some examples	Calories	Fat Grams	Fiber Grams
1 ounce, or about 3/4 cup, cereal (bran, oat, wheat flakes)	75-125	.5-1	2-5
1 bagel	200	1.5	1-2
1 English muffin	120	1	2
1 slice of most breads	60-80	1	2
1 6"-diameter pita bread	150	1	1-4
1/2 cup spaghetti or macaroni	100	.5	.5
1/2 cup whole wheat noodles	100	.5	3-4
1/2 cup rice (white, brown, wild, or various seasoned rice)	100-150	0-2	.5-2
1 flour tortilla	65	1	1
1 dinner roll	85	2	1

Comment: Most grain products are low in fat (typically well below 20 percent total calories), are good sources of fiber and the antioxidant vitamin E, and can improve insulin sensitivity. Notable exceptions to the low-fat rule are croissants and the average fat-laden muffin (though there are low-fat muffins on the market—you just have to be sure you get one). Choose products that say "whole wheat," "whole grain," or "enriched" on the label.

Vegetables (3-5 servings)

Serving size: 1/2 cup cooked or raw vegetables; 1 cup leafy vegetables; 3/4 cup vegetable juice.

Some examples	Calories	Fat Grams	Fiber Grams
1/2 cup carrots	25	trace	2
1/2 cup corn	80	"	4.5
1/2 cup spinach	6	"	1
1/2 cup squash	20-40	"	1.5-3
1 potato	150	"	4
1/2 cup sweet potatoes	100	"	4
1/2 cup tomatoes	15	"	1

Comment: Most vegetables have little, if any, fat in them (typically less than 5 percent of total calories), and they are excellent sources of fiber, antioxidants, and phytochemicals. Feel free to eat as many of them as you want. The more the better, probably, so no reason to hold back.

Fruits (2-4 servings)

Serving size: 1 average-sized piece of fruit; 1/2 grapefruit; 1/2 cup mixed fruit; 1/4 cup dried fruit; 3/4 cup fruit juice.

Some examples	Calories	Fat Grams	Fiber Grams
1 banana	100	trace	2
1 orange	65	"	4
1 apple	80	"	4
1 nectarine	70	"	3
1/2 grapefruit	40	"	1
1/2 cup melon	25-30	"	.5-1
1/2 cup strawberries	25	"	1.5
1/2 cup grapes	50	"	.5

1/4 cup dried fruit	90	"	2
3/4 cup orange juice	80	"	0

Comment: Like vegetables, most fruits have essentially no fat in them, and are also good sources of fiber, antioxidants, and phytochemicals. Feel free to eat as much fruit as you like—even more than the amounts recommended by the USDA. (The exceptions: avocados and coconuts—the latter technically a nut—which are very high in fat.)

Dairy: Milk, Yogurt, and Cheese (2-3 servings)

Serving size: 1 cup milk or yogurt; 1.5 ounces natural cheese; 2 ounces processed cheese.

Some Lower-Fat Choices	Calories	Fat Grams	Fiber Grams
1 cup 1%-fat milk	100	2.5	0
1 cup skim milk	85	.5	0
1 cup buttermilk	100	2	0
1 cup low-fat yogurt	140	4	0
1 cup nonfat yogurt	110	trace	0
1 cup reduced-fat or light cheese	60-80	4-5	0
Some Higher-Fat Choices			
1 cup whole milk	150	8	0
1 cup 2%-fat milk	120	5	0
1 cup whole-milk yogurt	150	7	0
1 ounce cheese (most)	80-120	6-9	0

Comment: Most dairy products are naturally high in fat, especially saturated fat. However, many low- and non-fat products are now on the market, which provide the same amount of nutrients (including calcium) but less of the fat. Keep in mind when reading food labels that the recommended daily intake of calcium is at least 1,000 milligrams (mg) per day (1,200 mg per day for women and men age 51 or older, with some research suggesting 1,500 mg per day for men over age 65 and for postmenopausal women not taking hormone replacement therapy). One cup of milk, regardless of fat content, contains about 300 mg calcium; 1 cup of yogurt between 300 and 400 mg; and 1 ounce of cheese between 150 and 250 mg.

Meat, Poultry, Fish, Dry Beans, Eggs, and Nuts (2-3 servings)

Serving size: 2 to 3 ounces cooked lean meat, poultry, or fish. A 3-ounce piece of meat, poultry, or fish will be about the size of a deck of playing cards. Also note that the following are equivalent to 1 ounce of meat: 1 egg, 2 tablespoons peanut butter, and 1/3 cup most nuts.

Some Examples	Calories	Fat Grams	Fiber Grams
3 ounces cooked ground beef			
90% lean (10% fat *by weight*)	193	10	0
79% lean (21% fat *by weight*)	252	18	0
3 ounces cooked top round steak			
"select" grade	155	4.5	0
"choice" grade	165	5.5	0
"prime" grade	185	7.5	0
3 ounces chicken			
Roasted:			
light meat, without skin	145	3	0
dark meat, without skin	155	5.5	0
Fried:			
light and dark, with skin	105-230	9-12	0
light and dark, without skin	175-195	5-8	0
3 ounces drained tuna			
water-packed	110	.5	0
oil-packed	170	7	0
3 ounces fish, most kinds, broiled or baked	90-110	1-2	0
3 ounces fatty fish (such as salmon and halibut), broiled or baked	150-160	6	0
1 egg	80	5.5	0
2 tablespoons peanut butter	190	16	2
1/3 cup mixed nuts	450	22	3
1/2 cup legumes (lentils, chick-peas, split peas, black beans, etc.)	90-150	0-1	4-8

Comment: You are better off limiting consumption of meat and eggs, and emphasizing poultry, fish, and dried beans (which, as legumes, can also be considered vegetables, but were listed in this group because of their high protein content). Most nuts are abundant in "good" fats; but be careful—calorie content is very high.

Fats, Oils, and Sweets

Some examples	Calories	Fat Grams	Fiber Grams
1 tablespoon:			
any oil (vegetable or animal)	120	14	0
butter	100	11	0
margarine	100	11	0
margarine (light)	60	6	0
mayonnaise	100	11	0
mayonnaise (light)	50	5	0
salad dressing	70-80	5-9	0
salad dressing (low calorie)	10-30	1-2	0
sweet roll, doughnut	150-250	8-12	1
1 ounce chocolate	150	8	0
1 cup ice cream			
gourmet	350	24	0
regular	270	14	0
1 cup frozen yogurt	200-250	0-4	0
1 slice fruit pie	400	15	3-4
1 slice pecan pie	600	30	2-3

Comment: It is best to use foods from this category sparingly. With regard to fats, as explained above, focus particularly on reducing your intake of saturated fats and hydrogenated and partially-hydrogenated vegetable oils (trans fats), but try to cut down on all fats. When you do use them, choose the oils that are high in monounsaturated fat (olive, canola, almond, and peanut) and/or polyunsaturated fat (corn, safflower, sesame, soybean, sunflower, walnut, and cottonseed), and avoid the ones that are high in saturated fat (coconut, palm, and palm kernel).

Looking at the Food Guide Pyramid and adding up the calories, you can begin to see how easy it could be to get close to 20 percent fat while still having a lot of flexibility in your food choices. If you eat from the bottom of the pyramid up, you'll note that 6 servings from "bread, cereal, rice and pasta," 2-4 servings of fruit, and 3-5 servings of vegetables will add up to about 1,000-1,200 calories and probably contain less than 10 grams of fat. If you're on a 2,000-calorie average daily total, that means you still have 800-1,000 calories you can add from the groups at the top, and about 34 grams of fat (out of the target total of 44). So you can put a little cream cheese on your bagel and butter or margarine on your English muffin. The milk doesn't have to be skim. The turkey-and-cheese sandwich can have some mayonnaise, and you'll still have room for a small helping of ice cream or some other fat- and sugar-laden goodie. Even if your "fatty" additions add up to 50 or even 55 grams per day on occasion, that will still correspond to less than 25 percent fat on 2,000 calories per day.

Tips on Reducing Fat in Your Diet

To show you how just a few simple changes can greatly reduce your consumption of fat, let's take a look at a hypothetical woman who eats 2,000 calories per day, 35 percent of which come from fat (700 calories or about 78 grams). Suppose 680 calories and 35 grams of fat out of the total come from 1 croissant (300 calories, 18 grams of fat), 2 cups of 2 percent fat milk (120 calories and 5 grams of fat in each cup), and a small scoop of regular ice cream (140 calories, 7 grams of fat).

If she exchanges her 2 percent fat milk for skim milk (85 calories, 0.5 grams of fat in each cup), the croissant for a bagel (200 calories, 1.5 grams of fat), and the ice cream for 2/3 cup frozen yogurt (140 calories, 2.5 grams of fat), she's down to 1,830 calories, 432 of which (48 grams) come from fat, for a total of about 23.6 percent. If she eats 3-4 additional servings of fruit or vegetables, for a total of about 170 calories and 1 gram of fat, she brings her total calorie consumption back up to 2,000, and her fat consumption of 441 calories (49 grams) now represents just 22 percent of the total. That's close enough to the target goal. But if she wants to get even lower, she can easily switch to nonfat frozen yogurt and get her fat percentage down to just under 21 percent.

Perhaps she doesn't like skim milk or nonfat frozen yogurt, or can't bear to give up her morning croissant. Other food exchanges that could be made to reduce fat consumption include the following: Instead of eating 6 ounces of breaded, skin-on chicken breasts (440 calories, 22 grams of fat), she could substitute chicken breasts without breading or skin (280 calories, 6 grams of fat) or 6 ounces of baked fish fillets (200 calories, 2 grams of fat). For a snack, she could eat 2/3 cup of pretzels (100 calories, no fat) or 1 ounce (13 chips) of baked tortilla chips (110 calories, 1 gram of fat) rather than 10 potato chips (105 calories, 7 grams of fat). On her dinner salad she could use 1 tablespoon of reduced-calorie dressing (25 calories, 2 grams of fat) rather than regular salad dressing (85 calories, 9 grams of fat). And so forth and so on. The key is to know which foods are high in fat, which ones are not, and to decide which of the high-fat ones you consider negotiable, which you feel you absolutely must hold on to.

If counting calories and keeping track of fat grams is just not for you, don't give up. Consult the following list for additional tips, and use as many of them as you can. Chances are you'll achieve a very substantial reduction in fat, even if you can't put a number to it.

- Have low-fat snack foods, especially fruits and vegetables, instantly available in the refrigerator. I recommend a bowl of fresh fruits—say a mix of apple, pear, and orange in the wintertime, strawberries, blueberries, peaches, and nectarines in the summer— and a jar full of cut-up fresh vegetables—say raw carrots, sugar snaps, broccoli, cauliflower, radishes, or whatever else suits you. If you wash, cut, peel, and chop the fruits and vegetables ahead of time, and store them in the refrigerator where they're ready for instant eating, you may go to them instead of to that bag of chips. Just take ten or fifteen minutes every few days to stock up your ready-to-eat fruit and veggie platters.

- Avoid fast-food restaurants. The quickest way to run up your tab on fat grams is to eat fast foods. The typical fast-food "entrée" has between 350 and 900 calories, and between 15 and 60 grams of fat. A Big Mac with a small serving of fries, for example, totals 820 calories and 43 grams of fat—practically a day's total fat allowance! A typical fast-food fish fillet will be 370-510 calories and 18-27 grams of fat. A taco salad at Taco Bell is 905 calories and 61 grams of fat! However, if you know how to choose carefully, you *can* find some relatively low-fat items—pizza among them—at the fast-food chains. Pizza, for example, depending on the topping, has between 150 and 250 calories and about 5-10 grams of fat per slice. You might want to consult one of the fast-food guides for suggestions for other food selections at places such as Wendy's, Kentucky Fried, Arby's, Burger King, McDonald's, and so forth.

- Choose many of the non- and low-fat versions of the items in the upper section of the Food Guide Pyramid (milk, yogurt, ice cream, salad dressings, and so on).

- Remove the skin from poultry before eating. Taking the skin from a half-breast of roasted chicken reduces the fat content from about eight grams to about three grams.

- Trim away all visible fat from meat. On a 3-ounce serving of sirloin steak, for example, this can reduce fat from 15 grams to 6 grams.

- Select only "lean" and "extra lean" meat (see discussion of food labels above). Try to think of meat as a side dish rather than the main course, and eat smaller portions of it, asking for the "petite" rather than the 12-ounce size in a restaurant, for example.

- Broil, roast, braise, steam, or poach your meat, fish, and poultry instead of frying them.

- Don't add oil when browning ground meats; do drain off the fat before mixing in other ingredients in a recipe using ground meat.

- Substitute jam, honey, or all-fruit, no-sugar-added preserves for butter or margarine on your toast.

- When preparing sauces, stuffing, or pasta, use only half or less of the butter, margarine, or olive oil called for in the recipe. You'll never know the difference.

- Whenever a recipe calls for milk or cream, use low-fat milk (such as 1 percent).

- Use egg whites instead of the whole egg in recipes.

- Get rid of your chips and cheese-loaded snacks and substitute low- or non-fat snack items such as pretzels, rice cakes, baked tortilla chips, and unbuttered popcorn.

- To minimize food sticking to pans, use vegetable-oil sprays to substitute for oil you pour out of a bottle. To avoid destroying the ozone, just keep, or buy, cooking oil in a spray-pump bottle.

- When dining out, look for these descriptions on the menu, which are almost always code for "high-fat": *buttered, French fried, breaded, cream fried, creamy, au gratin, scalloped, rich.* Gravies and hollandaise sauces, like most sauces in most restaurants, are high-fat. You can ask for the sauce to be omitted or put on the side.

Whether you follow any, or all, of these recommendations is up to you, but even a few of them can make a big difference; and remember that no foods are strictly off-limits. You can always balance your high-fat choices with other foods from the bottom half of the food pyramid. That's why I've placed at least as much emphasis on *adding* foods as on cutting them. Diversity is the key: A NHANES I follow-up survey that was carried out between 1982 and 1987 showed that those men and women who consumed two or fewer of the food groups—with deficiencies in fruits and vegetables being the most common—had mortality rates 40 to 50 percent higher than men and women who chose selections from all the food groups. Shockingly, only about three percent of U.S. citizens meet four of the five recommendations for the intake of grains, fruits, vegetables, dairy products, and meats.

Metabolic Fitness in a Pill?

In December, 1994, researchers at the Howard Hughes Medical Institute at Rockefeller University in New York reported that they had discovered and cloned a gene that regulates appetite and metabolism. Defective versions of the gene were discovered to be the factor responsible for extreme hereditary obesity in mice (hence its name, the "*ob* gene"). In its normal form the gene makes a protein that seems to tell the hypothalamus (the appetite-regulating part of the brain) when the body has had enough food and when to start burning off fat stores. The man who directed the research, Dr. Jeffrey Friedman, called this protein "leptin" (Greek for "thin").

When researchers injected leptin into the obese mice with the defective gene, the mice lost almost 30 percent of their body weight in two weeks. Even normal mice, when given the protein, lost nearly all of their body fat. When these results were published in the July 28, 1995, issue of *Science*, leptin was instantly heralded as a possible "cure" for obesity.

In light of the headline-making news about this magical "fat-burning hormone," perhaps you're thinking you can forget about exercise and low-fat, high-fiber foods and just wait for the "thin pill" to come along. After all, if a pill can make you thin, why bother to exercise? If a pill can burn off all the fat you eat that would otherwise be stored as body fat, why bother to cut fat from the diet? The answer to these questions depends on how body fat is viewed: as a cause of health problems, or as a symptom of unhealthy behaviors.

Regardless of how you view fat, the answer will also depend on whether this (or any other) protein can work in humans. With more than 3,000 studies on leptin published since its discovery in 1994 (yes, it did ignite a tremendous amount of interest!), the once-heralded "thin" protein has not lived up to the hype that accompanied its debut. The first clinical trial with leptin, published in the *Journal of the American Medical Association*, in 1999, provided mixed results. Low doses had virtually no effect, and even the highest dose produced widely varying responses: some subjects lost 20 pounds or more over 24 weeks of treatment, yet others actually *gained* weight! Thus, leptin may work for only an extremely small percentage of obese persons. Long-term efficacy is, however, unknown.

The initial experiments on the mice only lasted a month. When the mice went off leptin, they regained their appetite and their weight. For the relatively few humans for whom leptin might be helpful, will leptin have to be a lifelong medical regime? If so, what possible side effects could there be? And what about obesity that *isn't* a genetic problem? Would leptin exercise its appetite-lowering effects even on overeating that has nothing to do with real hunger? After all, it's lifestyle, not genes, that accounts for the roughly fifteen-pound increase in the average weight of U.S. adults, and the greatly increased prevalence of obesity, in the last 20 years or so. What effect can leptin have on lifestyle? Even though it works just fine on genetically obese mice living in the confines of a laboratory, can it override the effects of the thousands of TV commercials we see every year telling us to eat, eat, eat? Can it tell us to stop midway through a Whopper with cheese? Americans consume what might be called a "see" food diet. We see it, we want it. Can leptin defeat Madison Avenue? To believe that a pill is going to burn away the fat of the 118 million Americans who are considered overweight or obese by BMI standards is wishful thinking.

But what if it could? What if leptin—or any other weight-loss drug— did work, and we could all be thin by popping a pill? Will we stop all exercise, slip into total couch-potato-hood, and live on a diet of fast food, hot fudge sundaes, and candy? That's the direction we're headed, even without the promise of a magic pill. If exercise and nutrition are viewed merely as a means of achieving the single goal of thinness, then the "thin pill" may create a nation of *thin but unfit, unhealthy people.* Recall what happened to the cholesterol levels of people who tried the low-carbohydrate, high-fat diets for just a few weeks. Cholesterol went way up, even as weight was going down. Even more alarming are the research results from the Aerobics Center Longitudinal Study conducted by Dr. Steven Blair and his colleagues at the Cooper Institute, in Dallas, Texas. The thin, unfit men and women in this study were the people with the highest risk of premature death—death rates that were two or more times higher than the "fat but fit."

Throughout this century, we've been promised one "miracle cure" after another for obesity, and for the conditions caused by the lifestyle that leads to that obesity. What have they gotten us? An overdependence on pills to achieve what exercise and good nutrition could do at lower cost— to both our health and our pocketbooks. Take blood pressure medications, for example. In most cases high blood pressure could be effectively lowered with exercise and by reducing consumption of high-fat foods. Instead we take drugs, some of which create insulin resistance, thus causing one set of serious health problems at the same time that they are curing another. Exercise and a low-fat, high-fiber food plan, however, have no "side effects," and enhance rather than impair insulin sensitivity. Even when compared to medications that do improve insulin sensitivity, lifestyle changes seem to be more effective—as illustrated by the results of the landmark Diabetes Prevention Program, published in the February 7, 2002, issue of the *New England Journal of Medicine.*

Over a four-year period, 3,234 obese, nondiabetic men and women with elevated fasting glucose were assigned to either a control group, a drug group, or a lifestyle-modification group. The drug group received metformin (Glucophage®), an insulin sensitizing medication that helps lower blood glucose. The lifestyle-modification group was encouraged to lose at least seven percent of initial body weight via increasing physical activity (at least 150 minutes per week, or an average of about 21 minutes per day) and reducing fat intake. Although the lifestyle-modification participants were successful in upping their physical activity level and reducing fat intake (from 34.1 percent to 27.5 percent of total calories), at the four-year follow-up point, weight loss was only about 4 percent of initial body weight. Nevertheless the four-year incidence of diabetes in the lifestyle-modification group was reduced by 58 percent (compared to the control group), whereas the drug group experienced a 31 percent reduction in diabetes incidence. Though both interventions were effective, the authors of the study remarked that the "lifestyle intervention was more effective than metformin."

Science will never be able to create a drug to mimic every positive effect that exercise has been shown to have, nor a designer drug complete with the thousands of cancer-fighting phytochemicals contained in every fruit and vegetable. *Metabolic fitness can never be found in a pill.* It's still best to heed your mother's advice and eat your fruits and vegetables, and to exercise. As Hippocrates said, "Eating alone will not keep a man well; he must also take exercise. For food and exercise, while possessing opposite qualities, yet work together to produce health."

REFERENCES

Introduction

Ernsberger, P, and P Haskew. 1986. News about obesity. *N Engl J Med* 315: 130-131.

Gaesser, G. Nov. 10, 1997. Are the health risks of obesity exaggerated? *Insight*, pp. 24, 26-7.

Gaesser, GA. 1999. Thinness and weight loss: beneficial or detrimental to longevity? *Med Sci Sports Exerc* 31: 1118-1128.

Hutchinson, W. Aug. 21, 1926. Fat and Fashion. *Saturday Evening Post*, p. 58.

Chapter One

Fitzgerald, F. 1981. The problem of obesity. *Ann Rev Med* 32: 221-231.

Maiman, LA, VL Wang, MH Becker, T Finlay, and M Simonson. 1979. Attitudes toward obesity and the obese among professionals. *J Am Diet Assoc* 74: 331-336.

Perlmutter, C (with M Toth). Nov. 1994. Hitting your perfect weight. *Prevention*, pp. 65-73, 116-118.

Wadden, TA, and AJ Stunkard. 1985. Social and psychological consequences of obesity. *Ann Int Med* 103: 1062-1067.

Wooley, SC, and DM Garner. 1991. Obesity treatment: the high cost of false hope. *J Am Diet Assoc* 91: 1248-1251.

Diet Mania

Coakley, EH, EB Rimm, G Colditz, I Kawachi, and W Willett. 1998. Predictors of weight change in men: results from the Health Professionals Follow-up Study. *Int J Obes Relat Metab Disord* 22: 89-96.

French, SA, RW Jeffrey, JL Forster, PG McGovern, SH Kelder, and JE Baxter. 1994. Predictors of weight gain over two years among a population of working adults: the Healthy Worker Project. *Int J Obes Relat Metab Disord* 18: 145-154.

Grodstein, F, R Levine, L Troy, T Spencer, GA Colditz, and MJ Stampfer. 1996. Three-year follow-up of participants in a commercial weight loss program. Can you keep it off? *Arch Int Med* 156: 1302-1306.

Horn, J, and K Anderson. 1993. Who in America is trying to lose weight? *Ann Int Med* 119: 672-676.

Howard, L, and N Zeman. Feb. 3, 1992. Never on Sundae. *Newsweek*, p. 10.

Korkeila, M, A Rissanen, J Kaprio, TIA Sorensen, and M Koskenvuo. 1999. Weight-loss attempts and risk of major weight gain: a prospective study in Finnish adults. *Am J Clin Nutr* 70: 965-975.

Kuczmarski, RJ, KM Flegal, SM Campbell, and CL Johnson. 1994. Increasing prevalence of overweight among US adults: the National Health and Nutrition Examination Surveys, 1960-1991. *JAMA* 272: 205-211.

Mokdad, AH, BA Bowman, ES Ford, F Vinicor, JS Marks, and JP Koplan. 2001. The continuing epidemics of obesity and diabetes in the United States. *JAMA* 286: 1195-1200.

Mokdad, AH, MK Serdula, WH Dietz, BA Bowman, JS Marks, and JP Koplan. 1999. The spread of the obesity epidemic in the United States, 1991-1998. *JAMA* 282: 1519-1522.

NIH Technology Assessment Conference Panel. 1992. Methods for voluntary weight loss and control. *Ann Int Med* 116: 942-949.

Serdula, MK, ME Collins, DF Williamson, RF Anda, E Pamuk, and TE Byers. 1993. Weight control practices of US adolescents and adults. *Ann Int Med* 119: 667-671.

Serdula, MK, DF Williamson, RF Anda, A Levy, A Heaton, and T Byers. 1994. Weight control practices in adults: results of a multistate telephone survey. *Am J Pub Health* 84: 1821-1824.

Serdula, MK, AH Mokdad, DF Williamson, DA Galuska, JM Mendlein, and GW Heath. 1999. Prevalence of attempting weight loss and strategies for controlling weight. *JAMA* 282: 1353-1358.

Shapiro, L (with EA Leonard). May 13, 1991. Everybody's got a hungry heart. *Newsweek*, pp. 58-59.

Strauss, RS, and HA Pollack. 2001. Epidemic increase in childhood overweight, 1986-1998. *JAMA* 286: 2845-2848.

The American Society for Aesthetic Plastic Surgery. 2001 statistics charts and graphs. *www.surgery.org.*

Williamson, DF, MK Serdula, RF Anda, A Levy, and T Byers. 1992. Weight loss attempts in adults: Goals, duration, and rate of weight loss. *Am J Pub Health* 82: 1251-1257.

Defending Our Fat Supplies

Benini, ZL, MA Camilloni, C Scordato, et al. 2001. Contribution of weight cycling to serum leptin in human obesity. *Int J Obes Relat Metab Disord* 25: 721-726.

Coakley, EH, et al. 1998. Idem. *Int J Obes Relat Metab Disord* 22: 89-96.

de Zwann, M, and JE Mitchell. 1992. Binge eating in the obese. *Ann Med* 24: 303-308.

Drewnowski, A, C Kurth, J Holden-Wiltse, and J Saari. 1992. Food preferences in human obesity: Carbohydrates *versus* fats. *Appetite* 18: 207-221.

French, SA, et al. 1994. Idem. *Int J Obes Relat Metab Disord* 18: 145-154.

Glazer, G. 2001. Long-term pharmacotherapy of obesity 2000. A review of efficacy and safety. *Arch Int Med* 161: 1814-1824.

Keys, A, J Brozek, A Henschel, O Michelson, and H L Taylor. *Biology of Human Starvation.* 1950. Minnesota: Univ. Minnesota Press, pp. 126-129.

Korkeila, M, et al. 1999. Idem. *Am J Clin Nutr* 70: 965-975.

Leibel, RL, M Rosenbaum, and J Hirsch. 1995. Changes in energy expenditure resulting from altered body weight. *N Engl J Med* 332: 621-628.

Mauer, MM, RBS Harris, and TJ Bartness. 2001. The regulation of total body fat: lessons learned from lipectomy studies. *Neurosci Biobehav Rev* 25: 15-28.

Neel, JV. 1962. Diabetes mellitus: A "thrifty" genotype rendered detrimental by "progress"? *Am J Hum Genet* 14: 353-362.

Russell, C. Oct. 12, 1993. High cost of shedding pounds. *Washington Post,* Health News.

Winters, P. Dec. 12, 1988. *Ad Age,* p. 62

Other Costs and Consequences of Dieting

NIH Consensus Development Conference Statement. 1985. Health implications of obesity. *Ann Int Med* 103: 1073-1077.

Nelson, M, R Ash, C Mulvihill, TJ Peters, and P Rogers. 2001. Iron status, diet and cognitive function in British adolescent girls. *Proc Nutr Soc* 60 (Suppl 1): 59A.

Polivy, J, and CP Herman. 1985. Dieting and binging: a causal analysis. *Am Psychologist* 40: 193-201.

Chapter Two

Mann, GV. 1971. Obesity, the nutritional spook. *Am J Public Health* 61: 1491-1498.

Defining and Measuring Obesity

Barnard, RJ, EJ Ugianskis, DA Martin, and SB Inkeles. 1992. Role of Diet and exercise in the management of hyperinsulinemia and associated atherosclerotic risk factors. *Am J Cardiol* 69: 440-444.

Bennett, W, and J Gurin. 1982. *The Dieter's Dilemma: Eating Less and Weighing More.* New York: Basic Books, pp. 124-126.

Dublin, LI. 1989. *A Family of Thirty Million: The Story of the Metropolitan Life Insurance Company.* New York: MetLife, p. 17.

Ideal weights for women. Oct. 1942. *Stat Bull* 23: 2-8.

Ideal weights for men. June 1943. *Stat Bull* 24: 6-8.

National Heart, Lung, and Blood Institute. September 1998. Clinical guidelines on the identification, evaluation, and treatment of overweight and obesity in adults: the evidence report. NIH Publication No. 98-4083.

Rogers, OH. 1901. Build as a factor influencing longevity. *Association of Life Insurance Medical Directors of America,* 12th annual meeting, p. 280.

Seid, RP. 1989. *Never Too Thin: Why Women Are at War with Their Bodies.* New York: Prentice Hall, pp. 81-102.

Symonds, B. Jan. 1909. The mortality of overweights and underweights. *McClure's Magazine,* pp. 319-327.

Symonds, B. 1913-15. President's Address. *Association of Life Insurance Medical Directors of America,* 23rd-25th annual meetings, pp. 4-57.

"Overweight: America's Number-One Health Problem"

Armstrong, DB, LI Dublin, EC Bonnett, and HH Marks. 1951. Influence of overweight on health and disease. *Postgrad Med* 10: 407-422.

Chappell, R. July 23, 1956. The big bulge in profits. *Newsweek,* pp. 61-63.

Dublin, LI. July 1952. Stop killing your husband. *Reader's Digest,* pp. 107-109.

Dublin, LI, and HH Marks. 1937. The build of women and its relation to their mortality. A preliminary report. *Association of Life Insurance Medical Directors of America,* 48th annual meeting, pp. 47-85.

Dublin, LI. 1953. Relation of obesity to longevity. *N Engl J Med* 248: 971-974.

Obesity called waste of manpower and food. 1951. *Science Digest* 59: 377.

Obesity is now No. 1 US nutritional problem. 1952. *Science Digest* 62: 408.

The new American body. Dec. 1993. *University of California at Berkeley Wellness Letter.* 10: 1-2.

Zarrow, S (with C London). 1991. The new diet priorities. *Prevention*, pp. 33-36, 118-120.

Recommended Weights Drop Again

Build and Blood Pressure Study, 1959. 1960. Chicago: Society of Actuaries and Association of Life Insurance Medical Directors of America.

New weight standards for men and women. 1959. *Stat Bull* 40: 1-4.

The Antifat Movement

Bailey, C. 1978. *Fit or Fat?* Boston: Houghton Mifflin.

McArdle, WD, FI Katch, and VL Katch. 1996. *Exercise Physiology* (Fourth edition). Baltimore: Williams & Wilkins, pp. 570 and 608.

Pollock, ML, and JH Wilmore. 1990. *Exercise in Health and Disease* (Second edition). Philadelphia: W.B. Saunders, pp. 660-683.

Staying the Course

Brody, JE. Feb. 14, 1985. Panel terms obesity a major US killer needing top priority. *New York Times*, pp. A1, B8.

Build Study, 1979. 1980. Chicago: Society of Actuaries and Association of Life Insurance Medical Directors of America.

Kuczmarski, RJ, et al. 1994. Idem. *JAMA* 272: 205-211.

Manson, JE, WC Willett, MJ Stampfer, GA Colditz, DJ Hunter, SE Hankinson, CH Hennekens, and FE Speizer. 1995. Body weight and mortality among women. *N Engl J Med* 333: 677-685.

1983 Metropolitan Height and Weight Tables. 1983. *Stat Bull* 64: 2-9.

Mokdad, AH, et al. 1999. Idem. *JAMA* 282: 1519-1522.

Mokdad, AH, et al. 2001. Idem. *JAMA* 286: 1195-1200.

National Institutes of Health Consensus Development Conference Statement. 1985. Health implications of obesity. *Ann Int Med* 103: 1073-1077.

Rovner, S. Feb. 14, 1985. Obesity is 'killer disease' affecting 34 million Americans, NIH reports. *Washington Post,* p. 1.

What's your ideal weight? Oct. 1995. *Glamour*, pp. 250-253.

Chapter Three

Andres, R, D Elahi, JD Tobin, DC Muller, and L Brant. 1985. Impact of age on weight goals. *Ann Int Med* 103: 1030-1033.

Barrett-Connor, EL. 1985. Obesity, atherosclerosis, and coronary artery disease. *Ann Int Med* 103: 1010-1019.

Burton, BT, WR Foster, J Hirsch, and TB Van Itallie. 1985. Health implications of obesity: an NIH consensus development conference. *Int J Obesity* 9: 155-169.

Bjorntorp, P. 1985. Regional patterns of fat distribution. *Ann Int Med* 103: 994-995.

Dustan, HP. 1985. Obesity and hypertension. *Ann Int Med* 103: 1047-1049.

Iverius, P-H, and JD Brunzell. 1985. Obesity and common genetic metabolic disorders. *Ann Int Med* 103: 1050-1051.

Leibel, RL, and J Hirsch. 1985. Metabolic characterization of obesity. *Ann Int Med* 103: 1000-1002.

van Itallie, TB. 1985. Health implications of overweight and obesity in the United States. *Ann Int Med* 103: 983-988.

Obesity And Its Relationship to High Blood Pressure

Barrett-Connor, E, and K-T Khaw. 1985. Is hypertension more benign when associated with obesity? *Circulation* 72: 53-60.

Borkan, GA, D Sparrow, C Wisniewski, and PS Vokonas. 1986. Body weight and coronary disease risk: patterns of risk factor change associated with long-term weight change: the Normative Aging Study. *Am J Epidemiol* 124: 410-419.

Cambien, F, JM Chretien, P Ducimetiere, L Guize, and JL Richard. 1985. Is the relationship between blood pressure and cardiovascular risk dependent on body mass index? *Am J Epidemiol* 122: 434-442.

Carman, WJ, E Barrett-Connor, M Sowers, and K Khaw. 1994. Hypertensive/risk factors: higher risk of cardiovascular mortality among lean hypertensive individuals in Tecumseh, Michigan. *Circulation* 89: 703-711.

Ernsberger, P, and DO Nelson. 1988. Effects of fasting and refeeding on blood pressure are determined by nutritional state, not by body weight change. *Am J Hypertens* 1: 153S-157S.

Flegal, KM. 2000. Obesity, overweight, hypertension, and high blood cholesterol: the importance of age. *Obes Res* 8: 676-677.

Goldbourt, U, E Holtzman, L Cohen-Mandelzweig, and HN Neufeld. 1987. Enhanced risk of coronary heart disease mortality in lean hypertensive men. *Hypertension* 10: 22-28.

Guagnano, MT, V Pace-Palitti, C Carrabs, D Merlitti, and S Sensi. 1999. Weight fluctuations could increase blood pressure in android obese women. *Clin Sci* 96: 677-680.

Guagnano, MT, E Ballone, V Pace-Palitti, et al. 2000. Risk factors for hypertension in obese women. The role of weight cycling. *Eur J Clin Nutr* 54: 356-360.

Haynes, RB. 1986. Is weight loss an effective treatment for hypertension? The evidence against. *Can J Physiol Pharmacol* 64: 825-830.

Higgins, M, R D'Agostino, W Kannel, and J Cobb. 1993. Benefits and adverse effects of weight loss: observations from the Framingham Study. *Ann Int Med* 119: 758-763.

Messerli, FH. 1983. Cardiovascular adaptations to obesity and arterial hypertension: detrimental or beneficial? *Int J Cardiol* 3: 94-97.

Reisin, E, and HG Hutchinson. Obesity-hypertension: effects on the cardiovascular and renal system—the therapeutic approach. In: S Oparil and MA Weber, eds. 1999. *Hypertension*. Philadelphia: W.B. Saunders. pp. 206-210.

Schneider, RD, and FH Messerli. 1993. Does obesity influence early target organ damage in hypertensive patients? *Circulation* 87: 1482-1488.

Torgerson, JS, and L Sjostrom. 2001. The Swedish Obese Subjects (SOS) Study—rationale and results. *Int J Obes* 25 (Suppl): S2-S4.

Van Itallie, TB. 1985. Health implications of overweight and obesity in the United States. *Ann Int Med* 103: 983-988.

Wassertheil-Smoller, S, C Fann, RM Allman, et al. 2000. Relation of low body mass to death and stroke in the systolic hypertension in the elderly program. *Arch Int Med* 160: 494-500.

Weber, MA, JM Neutel, and DHG Smith. 2001. Contrasting clinical properties and exercise responses in obese and lean hypertensive patients. *J Am Coll Cardiol* 37: 169-174.

Weinsier, RL, RJ Fuchs, TD Kay, JH Triebwasser, and MC Lancaster. 1976. Body fat: its relationship to coronary heart disease, blood pressure, lipids and other risk factors measured in a large male population. *Am J Med* 61: 815-824.

Weinsier, RL, LD James, BE Darnell, HP Dustan, R Birch, and GR Hunter. 1991. Obesity-related hypertension: evaluation of the separate effects of energy restriction and weight reduction on hemodynamic and neuroendocrine status. *Am J Med* 90: 460-468.

What Autopsies Tell Us about Obesity and Atherosclerosis

Keys, A. 1954. Obesity and degenerative heart disease. *Am J Public Health* 44: 864-871.

McGill, HC, et al. 1968. General findings of the International Atherosclerosis Project. *Lab Invest* 18: 498-502.

Patel, YC, DA Eggen, and JP Strong. 1980. Obesity, smoking and atherosclerosis: a study of interassociations. *Atherosclerosis* 36: 481-490.

Warnes, CA, and WC Roberts. 1984. The heart in massive (more than 300 pounds or 136 kilograms) obesity: analysis of 12 patients studied at necropsy. *Am J Cardiol* 54: 1087-1091.

What Angiography Tells Us about Obesity and Atherosclerosis

Applegate, WB, JP Hughes, and RV Zwagg. 1991. Case-control study of coronary heart disease risk factors in the elderly. *J Clin Epidemiol* 44: 409-415.

Arntzenius, AC, et al. 1985. Diet, lipoproteins, and the progression of coronary atherosclerosis: the Leiden Intervention Trial. *N Engl J Med* 312: 805-811.

Blankenhorn, DH, RL Johnson, WJ Mack, HA El Zein, and LI Vailas. 1990. The influence of diet on the appearance of new lesions in human coronary arteries. *JAMA* 263: 1646-1652.

Kramer, JR, Y Matsuda, JC Mulligan, M Aronow, and WL Proudfit. 1981. Progression of coronary atherosclerosis. *Circulation* 63: 519-526.

What Ultrasound Tells Us about Obesity and Atherosclerosis

Chambless, LE, AR Folsom, V Davis, et al. 2002. Risk factors for progression of common carotid atherosclerosis: the Atherosclerosis Risk in Communities Study, 1987-1998. *Am J Epidemiol* 155: 38-47.

Salonen, T, and JT Salonen. 1990. Progression of carotid atherosclerosis and its determinations: a population-based ultrasonography study. *Atherosclerosis* 81: 33-40.

Weight and Its Relationship to Diabetes, Insulin Resistance, Blood Fat Levels, and Other Risk Factors for Heart Disease

Anderson, JW, and K Ward. 1979. High-carbohydrate, high-fiber diets for insulin-treated men with diabetes mellitus. *Am J Clin Nutr* 32: 2312-2321.

Appel, LJ, TJ Moore, E Obarzanek, et al. 1997. A clinical trial of the effects of dietary patterns on blood pressure. *New Engl J Med* 336: 1117-1124.

Barnard, RJ. 1991. Effects of life-style modification on serum lipids. *Arch Int Med* 151: 1389-1394.

Barnard, RJ, T Jung, and SB Inkeles. 1994. Diet and exercise in the treatment of NIDDM. *Diabetes Care* 17: 1469-1472.

Bjorntorp, P, K de Jounge, L Sjostrom, and L Sullivan. 1970. The effect of physical training on insulin production in obesity. *Metabolism* 19: 631-638.

de Lorgeril, M, S Renaud, N Mamelle, et al. 1994. Mediterranean alpha-linolenic acid-rich diet in secondary prevention of coronary heart disease. *Lancet* 343: 1454-1459.

Despres, J-P. 1993. Abdominal obesity as important component of insulin-resistance syndrome. *Nutrition* 9: 452-459.

Ehnholm, C, JK Huttunen, P Pietinen, et al. 1982. Effect of diet on serum lipoproteins in a population with a high risk of CHD. *New Engl J Med* 307: 850-855.

Fagard RH. 1999. Physical activity in the prevention and treatment of hypertension in the obese, *Med Sci Sports Exerc* 31 (Suppl): S624-S630.

Fukagawa, NK, JW Anderson, G Hageman, VR Young, and KL Minaker. 1990. High-carbohydrate, high-fiber diets increase peripheral insulin sensitivity in healthy young and old adults. *Am J Clin Nutr* 52: 524-528.

Hellenius, ML, I Krakau, and U de Faire. 1997. Favourable long-term effects from advice on diet and exercise given to healthy men with raised cardiovascular risk factors. *Nutr Metab Cardiovasc Dis* 7: 293-300.

Hypertension in the United States: 1960 to 1980 and 1987 estimates. 1989. *Stat Bull* 70: 13-17.

Lamarche, B, J-P Despres, M-C Pouliot, et al. 1992. Is body fat loss a determinant factor in the improvement of carbohydrate and lipid metabolism following aerobic exercise training in obese women? *Metabolism* 41: 1249-1256.

Leserman, J, EM Stuart, ME Mamish, et al. 1989. Nonpharmacologic intervention for hypertension: long-term follow-up. *J Cardiopulm Rehabil* 9: 316-324.

Reaven, G. 1988. Role of insulin resistance in human disease. *Diabetes* 37: 1595-1607.

Sacks, FM, LP Svetkey, WM Vollmer, et al. 2001. Effects on blood pressure of reduced dietary sodium and the dietary approaches to stop hypertension (DASH) diet. *New Engl J Med* 344: 3-10.

Sawicki, PT. 1992. General Discussion, p. 74 [Insulin Sensitivity: Cardioprotection vs. Metabolic Disorders]. *J Cardiovasc Pharmacol* 20 (Suppl 11): S1-S84.

Obesity Allegedly Kills 300,000 Americans Every Year: Where Is the Evidence?

American Dietetic Association. 1997. Position of the American Dietetic Association: weight management. *J Am Diet Assoc* 97: 71-74.

Manson, JE, and GA Faich. 1996. Pharmacotherapy for obesity—do the benefits outweigh the risks? *New Engl J Med* 335: 659-660.

McGinnis, JM, and WH Foege. 1993. Actual causes of death in the United States. *JAMA* 270: 2207-2212.

McGinnis, JM, and WH Foege. 1998. The obesity problem [letter]. *New Engl J Med* 338: 1157.

National Task Force on the Prevention and Treatment of Obesity. 1996. Long-term pharmacotherapy in the management of obesity. *JAMA* 276: 1907-1915.

A New Source for the 300,000 Figure—But Still No Evidence

Allison, DB, KR Fontaine, JE Manson, J Stevens, and TB VanItallie. 1999. Annual deaths attributable to obesity in the United States. *JAMA* 282: 1530-1538.

US Department of Health and Human Services. 2001. The Surgeon General's call to action to prevent and decrease overweight and obesity. Rockville, MD: US Department of Health and Human Services, Public Health Service, Office of the Surgeon General.

Chapter Four

Seid, RP. 1989. *Never Too Thin: Why Women Are at War with Their Bodies*. New York: Prentice Hall, p. 19.

Natural Weights

Bruch, H. 1957. *The Importance of Overweight*. New York: W.W. Norton & Co., pp. 57-73.

Must, A, J Spadano, EH Coakley, AE Field, G Colditz, and WH Dietz. 1999. The disease burden associated with overweight and obesity. *JAMA* 282: 1523-1529.

Polivy, J, and CP Herman. 1983. *Breaking the Diet Habit: The Natural Weight Alternative*. New York: Basic Books.

Fat and Fit

Barlow, CE, HW Kohl III, LW Gibbons, and SN Blair. 1995. Physical fitness, mortality and obesity. *Int J Obesity* 19 (Suppl 4): S41-S44.

Blair, SN, HW Kohl III, RS Paffenbarger, DG Clark, KH Cooper, and LW Gibbons. 1989. Physical fitness and all-cause mortality: a prospective study of healthy men and women. *JAMA* 262: 2395-2401.

Hopkins, PN, and RR Williams. 1981. A survey of 246 suggested coronary risk factors. *Atherosclerosis* 40: 1-52.

Lee, CD, SN Blair, and AS Jackson. 1999. Cardiorespiratory fitness, body composition, and all-cause and cardiovascular disease mortality in men. *Am J Clin Nutr* 69: 373-380.

Lee, CD, AS Jackson, and SN Blair. 1998. US weight guidelines: is it also important to consider cardiorespiratory fitness? *Int J Obes* 22 (Suppl 2): S2-S7.

Mokdad, AH, et al. 2001. Idem. *JAMA* 286: 1195-1200.

Paffenbarger, RS, RT Hyde, AL Wing, and C-C Hsieh. 1986. Physical activity, all-cause mortality, and longevity of college alumni. *N Engl J Med* 314: 605-613.

Seidell, JC, TLS Visscher, and RT Hoogeveen. 1999. Overweight and obesity in the mortality rate data: current evidence and research issues. *Med Sci Sports Exerc* 31 (Suppl): S597-S601.

Analyzing the Actuarial Data

Blackburn, H, and RW Parlin. 1966. Antecedents of disease. Insurance mortality experience. *Ann New York Acad Sci* 135: 965-1017.

Build and Blood Pressure Study, 1959. Chicago: Society of Actuaries and Association of Life Insurance Medical Directors of America.

Build and Blood Pressure Study, 1959. Idem.

Build Study, 1979. Chicago: Society of Actuaries and Association of Life Insurance Medical Directors of America. Idem.

Willett, WC, JE Manson, MJ Stampfer, GA Colditz, B Rosner, FE Speizer, and CH Hennekens. 1995. Weight, weight change, and coronary heart disease in women: risks within the "normal" weight range. *JAMA* 273: 461-465.

Williamson, DF. 1993. Descriptive epidemiology of body weight and weight change in US adults. *Ann Int Med* 119: 646-649.

Framingham Heart Study—1983 Report

Dannenberg, AL, JB Keller, PWF Wilson, and WP Castelli. 1989. Leisure time physical activity in the Framingham Offspring Study: description, seasonal variation, and risk factor correlates. *Am J Epidemiol* 129: 76-88.

Hubert, HB, M Feinleib, PM McNamara, WP Castelli. 1983. Obesity as an independent risk factor for cardiovascular disease: a 26-year follow-up of participants in the Framingham Heart Study. *Circulation* 67: 968-977.

Framingham Heart Study—1991 Report

Lissner, L, PM Odell, RB D'Agostino, JS Stokes III, BE Kreger, AJ Belanger, and KD Brownell. 1991. Variability of body weight and health outcomes in the Framingham population. *N Engl J Med* 324: 1839-1844.

Thinner *versus* Heavier: An Alternate View of the Evidence

Allison, DB, MS Faith, M Heo, D Townsend-Butterworth, and DF Williamson. 1999. Meta-analysis of the effect of excluding early deaths on the estimated relationship between body mass index and mortality. *Obes Res* 7: 342-354.

Andres, R. 1999. Beautiful hypotheses and ugly facts: the BMI-mortality association. *Obes Res* 7: 417-419.

Beaglehole, R, MA Foulkes, IA Prior, and EF Eyles. 1980. Cholesterol and mortality in New Zealand Maoris. *Br Med J* 280: 285-287.

Bengtsson, C, C Bjorkelund, L Lapidus, and L Lissner. 1994. Associations of serum lipid concentrations and obesity with mortality in women: 20-year follow up of participants in prospective population study in Gothenburg, Sweden. *Brit Med J* 307: 1385-1388.

Borhani, NO, HH Hechter, and L Breslow. 1963. Report of a ten-year follow-up study of the San Francisco Longshoreman. *J Chronic Dis* 16: 1251-1266.

Calle, EE, MJ Thun, JM Petrelli, C Rodriguez, and CW Heath. 1999. Body-mass index and mortality in a prospective cohort of US adults. *New Engl J Med* 341: 1097-1105.

Carmelli, D, J Halpern, GE Swan, A Dame, M McElroy, AB Gelb, and RH Rosenman. 1991. 27-year mortality in the Western Collaborative Group Study: construction of risk groups by recursive partitioning. *J Clin Epidemiol* 44: 1341-1351.

Cornoni-Huntley, JC, TB Harris, DF Everett, D Albanes, MS Micozzi, TP Miles, and JJ Feldman. 1991. An overview of body weight of older persons, including the impact on mortality: the National Health and Nutrition Examination Survey I—epidemiologic follow-up study. *J Clin Epidemiol* 44: 743-753.

Diehr, P, DE Bild, TB Harris, A Duxbury, D Siscovick, and M Rossi. 1998. Body mass index and mortality in nonsmoking older adults: the Cardiovascular Health Study. *Am J Pub Health* 88: 623-629.

Durazo-Arvizu, RA, DL McGee, RS Cooper, Y Liao, and A Luke. 1998. Mortality and optimal body mass index in a sample of the US population. *Am J Epidemiol* 147: 739-749.

Dorn, JM, EF Schisterman, W Kinkelstein, and M Trevisan. 1997. Body mass index and mortality in a general population sample of men and women. The Buffalo Health Study. *Am J Epidemiol* 146: 919-931.

Dyer, AR, J Stamler, DM Berkson, and HA Lindberg. 1975. Relationship of relative weight and body mass index to 14-year mortality in the Chicago Peoples Gas Company Study. *J Chronic Dis* 28: 109-123.

Ernsberger, P, and P Haskew. 1987. *Rethinking Obesity: An Alternative View of its Health Implications.* New York: Human Sciences Press.

Fontebonne, A, MA Charles, N Thibult, JL Richard, JR Claude, JM Warnet, GE Rosselin, and E Eschwege. 1991. Hyperinsulinemia as a predictor of coronary heart disease mortality in a healthy population: the Paris Prospective Study, 15-year follow-up. *Diabetologia* 34: 356-361.

Fried, P, RA Kronmal, AB Newman, et al. 1998. Risk factors for 5-year mortality in older adults. The Cardiovascular Health Study. *JAMA* 279: 585-592.

Gaesser, GA. 1999. Thinness and weight loss: beneficial or detrimental to longevity? *Med Sci Sports Exerc* 31: 1118-1128.

Garn, SM, VM Hawthorne, JJ Pilkington, and SD Pesick. 1983. Fatness and mortality in the West of Scotland. *Am J Clin Nutr* 38: 313-319.

Gordon, T, and JT Doyle. 1988. Weight and mortality in men: the Albany Study. *Int J Epidemiol* 17: 77-81.

Jarrett, RJ, MJ Shipley, and G Rose. 1982. Weight and mortality in the Whitehall Study. *Br Med J* 285: 535-537.

Grabowski, DC, and JE Ellis. 2001. High body mass index does not predict mortality in older people: analysis of the Longitudinal Study of Aging. *J Am Geriat Soc* 49: 968-979.

Hoes, AW, DE Grobbee, HA Valkenburg, J Lubsen, and A Hofman. 1993. Cardiovascular risk and all-cause mortality: a 12-year follow-up study in the Netherlands. *Eur J Epidemiol* 9: 285-292.

Ishii, T, Y Momose, H Esaki, and H Une. 1998. A prospective study on the relationship between body mass index and mortality in middle-aged and elderly people in Japan. *Jap J Pub Health* 45: 27-34.

Keil, JE, SE Sutherland, RG Knapp, DT Lackland, PC Gazes, and HA Tyroler. 1993. Mortality rates and risk factors for coronary disease in black as compared with white men and women. *N Engl J Med* 329: 73-78.

Keys, A, et al. 1985. Serum cholesterol and cancer mortality in the Seven Countries Study. *Am J Epidemiol* 121: 870-883.

Menotti, A, et al. 1993. Inter-cohort differences in coronary heart disease mortality in the 25-year follow-up of the Seven Countries Study. *Eur J Epidemiol* 9: 527-536.

Menotti, A, GC Descovich, M Lanti, A Spagnola, A Dormi, and F Seccareccia. 1993. Indexes of obesity and all-causes mortality in Italian epidemiological data. *Prev Med* 22: 293-303.

Pettitt, DJ, JR Lisse, WC Knowler, and PH Bennett. 1982. Mortality as a function of obesity and diabetes mellitus. *Am J Epidemiol* 115: 359-366.

Reynolds, MW, L Fredman, P Langenberg, and J Magaziner. 1999. Weight, weight change, and mortality in a random sample of older community-dwelling women. *J American Geriat* Soc 47: 1409-1414.

Rissanen, A, M Heliovaara, P Knekt, A Aromaa, and A Reunanen. 1989. Overweight and mortality in Finnish men. In: P Bjorntorp and S Rossner, ed. *Obesity in Europe 88*. Paris: John Libbey, pp. 61-68.

Rissanen, A, P Knekt, M Heliovaara, A Aromaa, A Reunanen, and J Maatela. 1991. Weight and mortality in Finnish women. *J Clin Epidemiol* 44: 787-795.

Seccareccia, F, M Lanti, A Menotti, and M Scanga. 1998. Role of body mass index in the prediction of all cause mortality in over 62,000 men and women. The Italian RIFLE Pooling Project. Risk Factor and Life Expectancy. *J Epidemiol Comm Health* 52: 20-26.

Shaper, AG, SG Wannamethee, and M Walker. 1997. Body weight: implications for the prevention of coronary heart disease, stroke, and diabetes mellitus in a cohort study of middle aged men. *Brit Med J* 314: 1311-1317.

Singh, PN, and KD Lindsted. 1998. Body mass and 26-year risk of mortality from specific diseases among women who never smoked. *Epidemiol* 9: 246-254.

Sorkin, JD, D Muller, and R Andres. 1994. Body mass index and mortality in Seventh-day Adventist men: a critique and re-analysis. *Int J Obes* 18: 752-754.

Stevens, J, JE Keil, PF Rust, HA Tyroler, CE Davis, and PC Gazes. 1992. Body mass index and body girths as predictors of mortality in black and white women. *Arch Int Med* 152: 1257-1262.

Stevens, J, JE Keil, PF Rust, RR Verdugo, CE Davis, HA Tyroler, and PC Gazes. 1992. Body mass index and body girths as predictors of mortality in black and white men. *Am J Epidemiol* 135: 1137-1146.

Troiano, RP, EA Frongillo, Jr, J Sobal, and DA Levitsky. 1996. The relationship between body weight and mortality: a quantitative analysis of combined information from existing studies. *Int J Obesity* 20: 63-75.

Tyroler, HA, MG Knowles, SB Wing, EE Logue, CE Davis, G Heiss, S Heyden, and CG Hames. 1984. Ischemic heart disease risk factors and twenty-year mortality in middle-aged Evans County black males. *Am Heart J* 108: 738-746.

Vandenbroucke, JP, BJ Mauritz, A de Bruin, JHH Verheesen, C van der Heide-Wessel, and RM van der Heide. 1984. Weight, smoking, and mortality. *JAMA* 252: 2859-2860.

Visscher, TLS, JC Seidell, A Menotti, et al. 2000. Underweight and overweight in relation to mortality among men aged 40-59 and 50-59 years: the Seven Countries Study. *Am J Epidemiol* 151: 660-666.

Wilcosky, T, J Hyde, JJB Anderson, S Bangdiwala, and B Duncan. 1990.

Obesity and mortality in the Lipid Research Clinics Program Follow-up Study. *J Clin Epidemiol* 43: 743-752.

Wienpahl, J, DR Ragland, and S Sidney. 1990. Body mass index and 15-year mortality in a cohort of black men and women. *J Clin Epidemiol* 43: 949-960.

Potential Health Benefits of Extra Pounds

Avioli, LV. 1991. Significance of osteoporosis: a growing international health care problem. *Calcif Tissue Int* 49 (Suppl): S5-S7.

Breslow, RA, R Ballard-Barbash, K Munoz, and BI Graubard. 2001. Long-term recreational physical activity and breast cancer in the National Health and Nutrition Examination Survey I Epidemiologic Follow-up Study. *Cancer Epidemiol Biomarkers Prev* 10: 805-808.

Colditz, GA, and B Rosner. 2000. Cumulative risk of breast cancer to age 70 years according to risk factor status: data from the Nurses' Health Study. *Am J Epidemiol* 152: 950-964.

Dawson-Hughes, B, C Shipp, L Sadowski, and G Dallal. 1987. Bone density of the radius, spine, and hip in relation to percent of ideal body weight in post-menopausal women. *Calcif Tissue Int* 40: 310-314.

Dirx, MJM, LE Voorrips, RA Goldbohm, and PA van den Brandt. 2001. Baseline recreational physical activity, history of sports participation, and postmenopausal breast carcinoma in the Netherlands Cohort Study. *Cancer* 92: 1638-1649.

Edelstein, SL, and E Barrett-Connor. 1993. Relation between body size and bone mineral density in elderly men and women. *Am J Epidemiol* 138: 160-169.

Felson, DT, Y Zhang, MT Hannan, and JJ Anderson. 1993. Effects of weight and body mass index on bone mineral density in men and women: the Framingham Study. *J Bone Min Res* 8: 567-573.

Garn, SM, K Rosenberg, and A Schaefer. 1983. Relationship between fatness level and size attainment in Central America. *Ecol Food Nutr* 13: 157-165.

Higgins, MW, JB Keller, M Becker, W Howatt, JR Landis, H Rotman, HG Wegman, and I Higgins. 1982. An index of risk for obstructive airway disease. *Am Rev Resp Dis* 125: 144-151.

Hooyman, JR, LJ Melton III, AM Nelson, WM O'Fallon, and BL Riggs. 1984. Fractures after rheumatoid arthritis: a population-based study. *Arth Rheumatism* 27: 1353-1361.

Hunter, DJ, and WC Willett. 1993. Diet, body size, and breast cancer. *Epidemiol Rev* 15: 110-132.

Kabat, GC, and EL Wynder. 1992. Body mass index and lung cancer risk. *Am J Epidemiol* 135: 769-774.

Kabat, GC. 1996. Aspects of the epidemiology of lung cancer in smokers and nonsmokers in the United States. *Lung Cancer* 15: 1-20.

Kohl, HW, JA Villegas, NF Gordon, and SN Blair. 1992. Cardiorespiratory fitness, glycemic status, and mortality risk in men. *Diabetes Care* 15: 184-192.

Landi, F, G Onder, G Gambassi, et al. 2000. Body mass index and mortality among hospitalized patients. *Arch Int Med* 160: 2641-2644.

London, SJ, GA Colditz, MJ Stampfer, WC Willett, B Rosner, and FE Speizer. 1989. Prospective study of relative weight, height, and risk of breast cancer. *JAMA* 262: 2853-2858.

Ribot, C, F Tremollieres, J-M Pouilles, M Bonneu, F German, and J-P Louvet. 1988. Obesity and postmenopausal bone loss: the influence of obesity on vertebral density and bone turnover in postmenopausal women. *Bone* 8: 327-331.

Seeman, E, LJ Melton III, WM O'Fallon, and BL Riggs. 1987. Risk factors for spinal osteoporosis in men. *Am J Med* 75: 977-983.

Shaper, AG, et al. 1997. Idem. *Brit Med J* 314: 1311-1317.

Shoff, SM, PA Newcomb, A Trentham-Dietz, et al. 2000. Early-life physical activity and postmenopausal breast cancer: effect of body size and weight change. *Cancer Epidemiol Biomarkers Prev* 9: 591-595.

Tremollieres, FA, J-M Pouilles, and C Ribot. 1993. Vertebral postmenopausal bone loss is reduced in overweight women: a longitudinal study in 155 early postmenopausal women. *J Clin Endocrinol Metab* 77: 683-686.

Tretli, S. 1989. Height and weight in relation to breast cancer morbidity and mortality: a prospective study of 570,000 women in Norway. *Int J Cancer* 44: 23-30.

Tverdal, A. 1986. Body mass index and incidence of tuberculosis. *Eur J Resp Dis* 69: 355-362.

US Dept of Health, Education and Welfare Pub. 1979. *Caloric and selected nutrient values for persons 1-74 years of age. First Health and Nutrition Examination Survey, United States, 1971-1974.* Pub. No. (PHS)-79-1657.

van den Brandt, PA, D Spiegelman, S-S Yaun, et al. 2000. Pooled analysis of prospective studies on height, weight, and breast cancer risk. *Am J Epidemiol* 152: 514-527.

Vatten, LJ, and S Kvinnsland. 1992. Prospective study of height, body mass index and risk of breast cancer. *Acta Oncologica* 31: 195-200.

Wardlaw, GM. 1993. Putting osteoporosis in perspective. *J Am Diet Assoc* 93: 1000-1006.

Chapter Five

Keys, A, 1980. Overweight, obesity, coronary heart disease and mortality. *Nutr Rev* 38: 297-307.

Weight Tables: Arbitrary, Random, and Meaningless

Andres, R, et al. 1985. Idem. *Ann Int Med* 103: 1030-1033.

Bryn Austin, S, and SL Gortmaker. 2001. Dieting and smoking initiation in early adolescent girls and boys: a prospective study. *Am J Pub Health* 91: 446-450.

Build Study, 1979, Idem, Tables D19 and D21, pp. 150, 152.

French, SA, CL Perry, GR Leon, and JA Fulkerson. 1994. Weight concerns, dieting behavior, and smoking initiation among adolescents: a prospective study. *Am J Public Health* 84: 1818-1820.

Knapp, TR. 1983. A methodological critique of the 'ideal weight' concept. *JAMA* 250: 506-510.

Individualized Ideal Body Weights and Set Points

Chumlea, WC, AF Roche, RM Siervogel, JL Knittle, and P Webb. 1981. Adipocytes and adiposity in adults. *Am J Clin Nutr* 343: 1798-1803.

Dietz, WH, and SL Gortmaker. 1985. Do we fatten our children at the television set? Obesity and television viewing in children and adolescents. *Pediatrics* 75: 807-812.

Harris, RB, 1990. Role of set-point theory in regulation of body weight. *FASEB J* 4: 3310-3318.

Keesey, RE, and TL Powley. 1986. The regulation of body weight. *Ann Rev Psychol* 37: 109-133.

Knittle, JL, K Timmers, F Ginsberg-Fellner, RE Brown, and DP Katz. 1979. The growth of adipose tissue in children and adolescents: cross-sectional and longitudinal studies of adipose cell number and size. *J Clin Invest* 63: 239-246.

Mauer, MM, et al. 2001. Idem. *Neurosci Biobehav Rev* 25: 15-28.

Oscai, LB, SP Babirak, FB Dubach, JA McGarr, and CN Spirakis. 1974. Exercise or food restriction: effect on adipose tissue cellularity. *Am J Physiol* 227: 901-904.

Sjostrom, L. Fat cells and body weight. In: AJ Stunkard, ed. 1980 *Obesity*. Philadelphia: Saunders, pp. 72-100.

The Fattening of America:
Set-Point Alteration and Weight Change

Astrup, A, B Buemann, NJ Christensen, and S Toubro. 1994. Failure to increase lipid oxidation in response to increasing dietary fat content in formerly obese women. *Am J Physiol* 266 (*Endocrinol Metab* 29): E592-E599.

Flatt, JP. 1987. Dietary fat, carbohydrate balance, and weight maintenance: effects of exercise. *Am J Clin Nutr* 45: 296-306.

Jequier, E. 1993. Body weight regulation in humans: the importance of nutrient balance. *NIPS* 8: 273-276.

Schutz, Y, A Tremblay, RL Weinsier, and KM Nelson. 1992. Role of fat oxidation in the long-term stabilization of body weight in obese women. *Am J Clin Nutr* 55: 670-674.

Body Fat Has Gotten a Bad Rap

Hutchinson, W. Aug. 21, 1926. Fat and Fashion. *Saturday Evening Post*, p. 58.

Chapter Six

Andres, R. 1980. Effect of obesity on total mortality. *Int J Obesity* 4: 381-386.

Pears and Apples

Brooks, JJ, and PM Perosio. Adipose tissue. In: SS Sternberg, ed. 1992. *Histology for Pathologists*. New York: Raven Press, pp. 33-60.

Freedman, DS, and AA Rim. 1989. The relation of body fat distribution, as assessed by six girth measurements, to diabetes mellitus in women. *Am J Public Health* 79: 715-720.

Hartz, AJ, DC Rupley, and AA Rimm. 1984. The association of girth measurements with disease in 32,856 women. *Am J Epidemiol* 119: 71-80.

Hunter, GR, T Kekes-Szabo, SW Snyder, C Nicholson, I Nyikos, and L Berland. 1997. Fat distribution, physical activity, and cardiovascular risk factors. *Med Sci*

Sports Exerc 29: 362-369.

Kissebah, AH, N Vydelingum, R Murray, DJ Evans, AJ Hartz, RK Kalkhoff, and PW Adams. 1982. Relation of body fat distribution to metabolic complications of obesity. *J Clin Endocrinol Metab* 54: 254-260.

Lemieux, S, D Prud'homme, C Bouchard, A Tremblay, and J-P Despres. 1993. Sex differences in the relation of visceral adipose tissue accumulation to total fatness. *Am J Clin Nutr* 58: 463-467.

Pouliot, M-C, et al. 1992. Visceral obesity in men: associations with glucose tolerance, plasma insulin, and lipoprotein levels. *Diabetes* 41: 826-834.

Rexrode, KM, VJ Carey, CH Hennekins, et al. 1998. Abdominal adiposity and coronary heart disease in women. *JAMA* 280: 1843-1848.

Seidell, JC, L Perusse, J-P Despres, and C Bouchard. 2001. Waist and hip circumferences have independent and opposite effects on cardiovascular disease risk factors: the Quebec Family Study. *Am J Clin Nutr* 74: 315-321.

Terry, RB, ML Stefanick, W Haskell, and PD Wood. 1991. Contributions of regional adipose tissue depots to plasma lipoprotein concentrations in overweight men and women: possible protective effects of thigh fat. *Metabolism* 40: 733-740.

Vague, J. 1947. La différenciation sexuelle, facteur déterminant des formes de l'obésité. *Presse Med* 30: 339-340.

Vague, J. 1956. The degree of masculine differentiation of obesities: a factor determining predisposition to diabetes, atherosclerosis, gout and uric calculus disease. *Am J Clin Nutr* 4: 20-28.

Visceral (or Deep) Abdominal Fat: The *Bad* Body Fat

Bouchard, C, J-P Despres, and P Mauriege. 1993. Genetic and nongenetic determinants of regional fat distribution. *Endocrine Rev* 14: 72-93.

A Lifestyle Recipe for Bad Body Fat

Barnard, RJ, and SJ Wen. 1994. Exercise and diet in the prevention and control of the metabolic syndrome. *Sports Med* 18: 218-228.

Barrett-Connor, E, and K-T Khaw. 1989. Cigarette smoking and increased central adiposity. *Ann Int Med* 111: 783-787.

Bosello, O, M Zamboni, F Armellini, and T Todesco. 1993. Biological and clinical aspects of regional body fat distribution. *Diab Nutr Metab* 6: 163-171.

Bjorntorp, P. 1991. Metabolic implications of body fat distribution. *Diabetes Care* 14: 1132-1143.

Bjorntorp, P. 1988. The associations between obesity, adipose tissue distribution and disease. *Acta Med Scand Suppl* 273: 121-134.

Jayo, JM, CA Shively, JR Kaplan, and SB Manuck. 1993. Effects of exercise and stress on body fat distribution in male cynomolgus monkeys. *Int J Obesity* 17: 597-604.

Matsuzawa, Y, I Shimomura, T Nakamura, Y Keno, and K Tokunaga. 1993. Pathophysiology and pathogenesis of visceral fat obesity. *Ann New York Acad Sci* 676: 270-278.

Wing, RR, KA Matthews, LH Kuller, EN Meilahn, and P Plantinga. 1991. Waist to hip ratio in middle-aged women: associations with behavioral and psychosocial factors and with changes in cardiovascular risk factors. *Arteriosclerosis Thromb* 11: 1250-1257.

Subcutaneous Fat: The Good Body Fat

Berntorp, E, K Berntorp, H Brorson, and K Frick. 1998. Liposuction in Dercum's disease: impact on haemostatic factors associated with cardiovascular disease and insulin sensitivity. *J Int Med* 243: 197-201.

Eckel, RH, and TJ Yost. 1987. Weight reduction increases adipose tissue lipoprotein lipase responsiveness in obese women. *J Clin Invest* 80: 992-997.

Giese, S, EJ Bulan, GW Commons, SL Spear, and JA Yanovski. 2001. Improvements in cardiovascular risk profile with large-volume liposuction: a pilot study. *Plast Reconstr Surg* 108: 510-519.

Grazer, FM, and RH de Jong. 2000. Fatal outcomes from liposuction: census survey of cosmetic surgeons. *Plast Reconstr Surg* 105: 436-446.

Kral, JG. 1975. Surgical reduction of adipose tissue hypercellularity in man. *Scand J Plast Reconstr Surg* 9: 140-143.

Kral, JG, and LV Sjostrom. Surgical reduction of adipose tissue hypercellularity. In: A Howard, ed. 1975. *Recent Advances in Obesity Research: I.* London: Newman Publishing, pp. 327-330.

Kral, JG. 1988. Surgical treatment of regional adiposity: lipectomy *versus* surgically induced weight loss. *Acta Med Scand* 723 (Suppl): 225-231.

Larson, KA, and DB Anderson. 1978. The effects of lipectomy on remaining adipose tissue depots in the Sprague-Dawley rat. *Growth* 42: 469-477.

Matarasso, A, RW Kim, and J Kral. 1998. The impact of liposuction of body fat. *Plast Reconstr Surg* 102: 1686-1689.

Weber, RV, MC Buckley, SK Fried, and JG Kral. 2000. Subcutaneous lipectomy causes a metabolic syndrome in hamsters. *Am J Physiol Regulatory Integrative Comp Physiol* 279: R936-R943.

Are You an Apple or a Pear?

Bengtsson, C, et al. 1994. Idem. *Brit Med J* 307: 1385-1388.

Bray, GA. 1992. Pathophysiology of obesity. *Am J Clin Nutr* 55: 488S-494S.

Lapidus, L, C Bengtsson, B Larsson, K Pennert, E Rybo, and L Sjostrom. 1984. Distribution of adipose tissue and risk of cardiovascular disease and death: a 12-year follow up of participants in the population study of women in Gothenburg, Sweden. *Br Med J* 289: 1257-1261.

Larsson, B, K Svardsudd, L Welin, L Wilhelmsen, P Bjorntorp, and G Tibblin. 1984. Abdominal adipose tissue distribution, obesity, and risk of cardiovascular disease and death: 13-year follow up of participants in the study of men born in 1913. *Br Med J* 288: 1401-1404.

National Heart, Lung, and Blood Institute. September 1998. Idem. NIH Publication No. 98-4083.

Pouliot, M-C, J-P Despres, S Lemieux, et al. 1994. Waist circumference and abdominal sagittal diameter: best simple anthropometric indexes of abdominal visceral adipose tissue accumulation and related cardiovascular risk in men and women. *Am J Cardiol* 73: 460-468.

How to Interpret Your Measurments

Lee, CD, et al. 1999. Idem. *Am J Clin Nutr* 69: 373-380.

Chapter Seven

Kassirer, JP, and M Angell. 1998. Losing weight: an ill-fated New Year's resolution. *New Engl J Med* 338: 52-54.

Kuczmarski, RJ, et al. 1994. Idem. *JAMA* 272: 205-211.

Mokdad, AH, et al. 1999. Idem. *JAMA* 282: 1519-1522.

Serdula, MK, et al. 1999. Idem. *JAMA* 282: 1353-1358.

Williamson, DF, et al. 1992. Idem, *Am J Pub Health* 82: 1251-1257.

Evidence Refutes the Weight Loss Panacea

Andres, R, DC Muller, and JD Sorkin. 1993. Long-term effects of change in body weight on all-cause mortality: a review. *Ann Int Med* 119: 737-743.

Blair, SN, J Shaten, K Brownell, G Collins, and L Lissner. 1993. Body weight change, all-cause mortality, and cause-specific mortality in the Multiple Risk Factor Intervention Trial. *Ann Int Med* 119: 749-757.

Dyer, AR, J Stamler, and P Greenland. 2000. Associations of weight change and weight variability with cardiovascular and all-cause mortality in the Chicago Western Electric Company Study. *Am J Epidemiol* 152: 324-333.

Gaesser, GA. 1999. Idem. *Med Sci Sports Exerc* 31: 1118-1128.

Galanis, DJ, T Harris, DS Sharp, and H Petrovich. 1998. Relative weight, weight change, and risk of coronary heart disease in the Honolulu Heart Program. *Am J Epidemiol* 147: 379-386.

Harris, TB, R Ballard-Barbasch, J Madans, DM Makuc, and JJ Feldman. 1993. Overweight, weight loss, and risk of coronary heart disease in older women: the NHANES I Epidemiologic Follow-up Study. *Am J Epidemiol* 137: 1318-1327.

Higgins, M, et al. 1993. Idem. *Ann Int Med* 119: 758-763.

Lee, I-M, and RS Paffenbarger. 1992. Change in body weight and longevity. *JAMA* 268: 2045-2049.

Pamuk, ER, DF Williamson, J Madans, MK Serdula, JC Kleinman, and T Byers. 1992. Weight loss and mortality in a national cohort of adults, 1971-1987. *Am J Epidemiol* 136: 686-697.

Pamuk, ER, DF Williamson, MK Serdula, J Madans, and TE Byers. 1993. Weight loss and subsequent death in a cohort of US adults. *Ann Int Med* 119: 744-748.

Reynolds, MW, L Fredman, P Langenberg, and J Magaziner. 1999. Idem. *J American Geriat Soc* 47: 1409-1414.

Singh, PN, and KD Lindsted. 1998. Idem. *Epidemiol* 9: 246-254.

Wannamethee, SG, AG Shaper, and M Walker. 2001. Weight change, body weight and mortality: the impact of smoking and ill health. *Int J Epidemiol* 30: 777-786.

Williamson, DF, and ER Pamuk. 1993. The association between weight loss and increased longevity: a review of the evidence. *Ann Int Med* 119: 731-736.

Woo, J, SC Ho, and A Sham. 2001. Longitudinal changes in body mass index and body composition over 3 years and relationship to health outcomes in Hong Kong Chinese age 70 and older. *J American Geriat Soc* 49: 737-746.

Unintentional Weight Loss Cannot Explain the Findings

Diehr, P, et al. 1998. Idem. *Am J Pub Health* 88: 623-629.

French, SA, AR Folsom, RW Jeffrey, and DF Williamson. 1999. Prospective study of intentionality of weight loss and mortality in older women: the Iowa Women's Health Study. *Am J Epidemiol* 149: 504-514.

Hammond, EC, and L Garfinkel. 1969. Coronary heart disease, stroke, and aortic aneurysm. *Arch Environ Health* 19: 167-182.

Williamson, DF, E Pamuk, M Thun, D Flanders, T Byers, and C Heath. 1995. Prospective study of intentional weight loss and mortality in never-smoking overweight US white women aged 40-64 years. *Am J Epidemiol* 141: 1128-1141.

Williamson, DF, E Pamuk, M Thun, D Flanders, T Byers, and C Heath. 1999. Prospective study of intentional weight loss and mortality in overweight white men aged 40-64 years. *Am J Epidemiol* 149: 491-503.

The Weight Loss Paradox: Yo-Yoing to Death

Blair, SN, and RS Paffenbarger. March 16-19, 1994. Influence of body weight and shape variation on incidence of cardiovascular disease, diabetes, lung disease, and cancer. Harvard Alumni data: paper presented at the 34th Annual Conference on Cardiovascular Disease Epidemiology and Prevention.

Blair, SN, et al. 1993. Idem. *Ann Int Med* 119: 749-757.

Hamm, P, RB Shekelle, and J Stamler. 1989. Large fluctuations in body weight during young adulthood and twenty-five-year risk of coronary death in men. *Am J Epidemiol* 129: 312-318.

Holbrook, TL, E Barrett-Connor, and DL Wingard. 1989. The association of lifetime weight and weight control patterns with diabetes among men and women in an adult community. *Int J Obesity* 13: 723-729.

Iribarren, C, DS Sharp, CM Burchfiel, and H Petrovich. 1995. Association of weight loss and weight fluctuation with mortality among Japanese American men. *N Engl J Med* 333: 686-692.

Lee, I-M, and RS Paffenbarger, 1992. Idem. *JAMA* 268: 2045-2049.

Lissner, L, C Bengtsson, L Lapidus, B Larsson, B Bengtsson, and K Brownell. Body weight variability and mortality in the Gothenburg prospective studies of men and women. In: P Bjorntorp and S Rössner, eds. 1989. *Obesity in Europe 88*. London: John Libbey, pp. 55-60.

Lissner, L, et al. 1991. Idem. *N Engl J Med* 324: 1839-1844.

National Task Force on the Prevention and Treatment of Obesity. Weight Cycling. 1994. *JAMA* 272: 1196-1202.

Personal communication with SN Blair.

Lessons from Leningrad, Minnesota, and the Laboratory

Brozek, J, CB Chapman, and A Keys. 1948. Drastic food restriction: effect on cardiovascular dynamics in normotensive and hypertensive conditions. *JAMA* 137: 1569-1574.

Chen, Z-Y, M-M Sea, K-Y Kwan, Y-H Leung, and P-F Leung. 1997. Depletion of linoleate induced by weight cycling is independent of extent of calorie restriction. *Am J Physiol* 272 *(Regulatory Integrative Comp Physiol* 41*)*: R43-R50.

Ernsberger, P, and RJ Koletsky. 1993. Weight cycling and mortality: support from animal studies. *JAMA* 269: 1116.

Ernsberger, P, RJ Koletsky, JS Baskin, and LA Collins. 1996. Consequences of weight cycling in obese spontaneously hypertensive rats. *Am J Physiol* 270 *(Regulatory Integrative Comp Physiol* 39): R864-R872.

Ernsberger, P, and DO Nelson. 1988. Refeeding hypertension in dietary obesity. *Am J Physiol* 254 *(Regulatory Integrative Comp Physiol* 23*)*: R47-R55.

Ernsberger, P, and DO Nelson. 1988. Idem. *Am J Hypertens* 1: 153S-157S.

Gaesser, GA. 1999. Idem. *Med Sci Sports Exerc* 31: 1118-1128.

Guagnano, MT, et al. 1999. Idem. *Clin Sci* 96: 677-680.

Guagnano, MT, et al. 2000. Idem. *Eur J Clin Nutr* 54: 356-360.

Hembrough, FB, and DH Riedesel. 1970. Mechanical behavior change in a major artery after a series of starvation-refeeding episodes. *Am J Physiol* 219: 742-746.

Hewing, R, H Liebermeister, H Daweke, FA Gries, and D Gruneklee. 1973. Weight regain after low calorie diet: long term pattern of blood sugar, serum lipids, ketone bodies and serum insulin levels. *Diabetalogia* 9: 197-202.

Kajioka, T, S Tsuzuki, H Shimokata, and Y Sato. 2002. Effects of intentional weight cycling on non-obese young women. *Metabolism* 51: 149-154.

Keys, A, J Brozek, A Henschel, O Michelson, and H Longhurst. 1950. *Biology of Human Starvation*. Minnesota: Univ. of Minnesota Press, pp. 618-622.

Levin, BE. 1994. Diet cycling and age alter weight gain and insulin levels in rats. *Am J Physiol* 267 *(Regulatory Integrative Comp Physiol* 36*)*: R527-R535.

Pfohl, M, D Luft, I Blumberg, and R-M Schmilling. 1994. Long-term changes of body weight and cardiovascular risk factors after weight reduction with group therapy and dexfenfluramine. *Int J Obes* 18: 391-395.

Phinney, SD. 1992. Weight cycling and cardiovascular risk in obese men and women. *Am J Clin Nutr* 56: 781.

Phinney, SD, AB Tang, SB Johnson, and RT Holman. 1990. Reduced adipose 18:3w3 with weight loss by very low calorie dieting. *Lipids* 25: 798-806.

Sea, M-M, WP Fong, Y Huang, and Z-Y Chen. 2000. Weight cycling-induced alteration in fatty acid metabolism. *Am J Physiol Regulatory Integrative Comp Physiol* 279: R1145-R1155.

Smith, GS, JL Smith, MS Mameesh, J Simon, and BC Johnson. 1964. Hypertension and cardiovascular abnormalities in starved-refed swine. *J Nutrition* 82: 173-182.

Smith-Vaniz, GT, AD Ashburn, and WL Williams. 1970. Diet-induced hypertension and cardiovascular lesions in mice. *Yale J Biol Med* 43: 61-69.

Tang, AB, KY Nishimura, and SD Phinney. 1993. Preferential reduction in adipose tissue a-linolenic acid (18:3w3) during very low calorie dieting despite supplementation with 18:3w3. *Lipids* 28: 987-993.

US Public Health Service. 1966. *Obesity and Health*. Publication No. 1485. Washington D.C.: US Government Printing Office, p. 40.

Wilhelmj, CM, AJ Carnazzo, and HH McCarthy. 1957. Effect of fasting and realimentation with diets high in carbohydrate or protein on blood pressure and heart rate of sympathectomized dogs. *Am J Physiol* 191: 103-107.

The Low-Carbohydrate Way to Heart Disease

Cleland, JGF, and DM Krikler. 1993. Modification of atherosclerosis by agents that do not lower cholesterol. *Br Heart J* 69 (Suppl): S54-S62.

LaRosa, JC, AG Fry, R Muesing, and DR Rosing. 1980. Effects of high-protein, low-carbohydrate dieting on plasma lipoproteins and body weight. *J Am Diet Assoc* 77: 264-270.

Rickman, F, N Mitchell, J Dingman, and JE Dalen. 1974. Changes in serum cholesterol during the Stillman Diet. *JAMA* 228: 54-58.

Dieting Begets Bingeing, Which Begets...

Drewnowski, A, and J Holden-Wiltse. 1992. Taste responses and food preferences in obese women: effects of weight cycling. *Int J Obesity* 16: 639-648.

Garner, DM, and SC Wooley. 1991. Confronting the failure of behavioral and dietary treatments for obesity. *Clin Psychol Rev* 11: 729-780.

Grodstein, F. 1996. Idem. *Arch Int Med* 156: 1302-1306.

Hewing, R, et al. 1973. Idem. *Diabetalogia* 9: 197-202.

Ikeda, JP, D Hayes, E Satter, et al. 1999. A commentary on the new obesity guidelines from NIH. *J Am Diet Assoc* 99: 918-919.

NIH Technology Assessment Conference Panel. 1992. Idem. *Ann Int Med* 116: 942-949

Olson, MB, SF Kelsey, V Bittner, et al. 2000. Weight cycling and high-density lipoprotein cholesterol in women: evidence of an adverse effect. *J Amer Coll Cardiol* 36: 1565-1571.

Pfohl, M, et al. 1994. Idem. *Int J Obes* 18: 391-395.

Polivy, J, and CP Herman, 1985. Idem. *Am Psychologist* 40: 193-201.

Dieter's Dilemma: The Risk-*versus*-Benefit Analysis

Bates, GW. 1985. Body weight control practice as a cause of infertility. *Clin Obstet Gynecol* 28: 632-644.

Bennett, W, and J Gurin. 1982. *The Dieter's Dilemma.* Idem, p. 114.

Berg, FM. 1999. Health risks associated with weight loss and obesity treatment programs. *J Soc Issues* 55: 277-297.

Connoly, HM, JL Crary, MD McGoon, et al. 1997. Valvular heart disease associated with fenfluramine-phentermine. *New Engl J Med* 337: 581-588.

Curfman, GD. 1997. Diet Pills Redux. *New Engl J Med* 337: 629-630.

Djuric, Z, LK Heilbrun, S Lababidi, E Berzinkas, MS Simon, and MA Kosir. 2001. Levels of 5-hydroxymethyl-2'-deoxyuridine in DNA from blood of women scheduled for breast biopsy. *Cancer Epidemiol Biomarkers Prev* 10: 147-149.

Ernsberger, P, and P Haskew. 1987. *Rethinking Obesity: An Alternative View of its Health Implications.* New York: Human Sciences Press.

Fogelholm, M, H Sievanen, A Heinonen, et al. 1997. Association between weight cycling history and bone mineral density in premenopausal women. *Osteo Int* 7: 354-358.

Haller, CA, and NL Benowitz. 2000. Adverse cardiovascular and central nervous system events associated with dietary supplements containing ephedra alkaloids. *New Engl J Med* 343: 1833-1838.

Hill, AJ. 1993. Pre-adolescent dieting: implications for eating disorders. *Int Rev Psych* 5: 87-100.

Holbrook, TL, and E Barrett-Connor. 1993. The association of lifetime weight and weight control patterns with bone mineral density in an adult community. *Bone and Mineral* 20: 141-149.

Kernan, WN, CM Viscoli, LM Brass, et al. 2000. Phenylpropanolamine and the risk of hemorrhagic stroke. *New Engl J Med* 343: 1826-1832.

Lindblad, P, A Wolk, R Bergstrom, I Persson, and HO Adami. 1994. The role of obesity and weight fluctuations in the etiology of renal cell cancer: a population-based case-control study. *Cancer Epidemiol Biomarkers Prev* 3: 631-639.

Mark, EJ, ED Patalas, HT Chang, RJ Evans, and SC Kessler. 1997. Fatal pulmonary hypertension associated with short-term use of fenfluramine and phentermine. *New Engl J Med* 337: 602-606.

Polivy, J. 1996. Psychological consequences of food restriction. *J Am Diet Assoc* 96: 589-592.

Serdula, MK, et al. 1999. Idem. *JAMA* 282: 1353-1358.

Syngal S, EH Coakley, WC Willett, T Byers, DF Williamson, and GA Colditz. 1999. Long-term weight patterns and risk for cholecystectomy in women. *Ann Int Med* 130: 471-477.

Tagliaferro, AR, AM Ronan, LD Meeker, HJ Thompson, AL Scott, and D Sinha. 1996. Cyclic food restriction alters substrate utilization and abolishes protection from mammary carcinogenesis in female rats. *J Nutr* 126: 1398-1405.

Uhley, VE, MA Pellizzon, AM Buison, F Guo, Z Djuric, and K-L C Jen. 1997. Chronic weight cycling increases oxidative DNA damage levels in mammary gland of female rats fed a high-fat diet. *Nutr Cancer* 29: 55-59.

Vigersky, RA, AE Andersen, RH Thompson, and DL Loriaux. 1977. Hypothalamic dysfunction in secondary amenorrhea associated with simple weight loss. *N Engl J Med* 297: 1141-1145.

Who Pays the Price, and How High Is It?

Drenick, EJ, GS Bale, F Seltzer, and DG Johnson. 1980. Excessive mortality and causes of death in morbidly obese men. *JAMA* 243: 443-445.

Johnson, D, and EJ Drenick. 1977. Therapeutic fasting in morbid obesity. *Arch Int Med* 137: 1381-1382.

Chapter Eight

ACSM position stand on the recommended quantity and quality of exercise for developing and maintaining cardiorespiratory and muscular fitness, and flexibility in healthy adults. 1998. *Med Sci Sports Exerc* 30: 975-991.

Campfield, LA, FJ Smith, and P Burn. 1998. Strategies and potential molecular targets for obesity treatment. *Science* 280: 1383-1387.

Ernsberger, P, and P Haskew. 1986. News about obesity. *N Engl J Med* 315: 130-131.

US Dept Of Health and Human Services. 1996. *Physical Activity and Health: A Report of the Surgeon General.* Atlanta, GA: US Dept Of Health and Human Services, Centers for Disease Control and Prevention, National Center for Chronic Disease Prevention and Health Promotion.

Williamson, DF, et al. 1992. Idem. *Am J Public Health* 82: 1251-1257.

What It Means to Be Metabolically Fit: Insulin Sensitivity

Barnard, RJ, and SJ Wen. 1994. Idem. *Sports Med* 18: 218-228.

Barnard, RJ, JF Youngren, and DA Martin. 1995. Diet, not aging, causes skeletal muscle insulin resistance. *Gerontology* 41: 205-211.

Despres, J-P, B Lamarche, P Mauriege, et al. 1996. Hyperinsulinemia as an independent risk factor for ischemic heart disease. *New Engl J Med* 334: 952-957.

Despres, J-P. 1993. Idem. *Nutrition* 9: 452-459.

Ducimetiere, P, E Eschwege, L Papoz, JL Richard, JR Claude, and G Rosselin. 1980. Relationship of plasma insulin levels to the incidence of myocardial infarction and coronary heart disease mortality. *Diabetologia* 19: 205-210.

Ford, ES, WH Giles, and WH Dietz. 2002. Prevalence of the metabolic syndrome among US adults. *JAMA* 287: 356-359.

Kaplan, NM. 1989. The deadly quartet: upper-body obesity, glucose intolerance, hypertriglyceridemia, and hypertension. *Arch Int Med* 149: 1514-1520.

Martin, BC, JH Warram, AS Krolewski, RN Bergman, JS Soeldner, and CR Kahn. 1992. Role of glucose and insulin resistance in development of type 2 diabetes mellitus: results of a 25-year follow-up study. *Lancet* 340: 925-929.

Reaven, GM. Idem. *Diabetes* 37: 1595-1607.

Yam, D. 1992. Insulin-cancer relationships: possible dietary implication. *Med Hypoth* 38: 111-117.

Are You Insulin Resistant?

Executive summary of the Third Report on the National Cholesterol Education Program (NCEP) Expert Panel on Detection, Evaluation, and Treatment of High Blood Cholesterol in Adults (Adult Treatment Panel III). 2001. *JAMA* 285: 2486-2497.

Causes of Insulin Resistance: Genes and Beyond

Barker, DJP, CN Hales, CHD Fall, C Osmond, K Phipps, and PMS Clark. 1993. Type 2 (non-insulin-dependent) diabetes mellitus, hypertension and hyperlipidemia (syndrome X): relation to reduced fetal growth. *Diabetologia* 36: 62-67.

Egusa, G, et al. 1993. Westernized food habits and concentrations of serum lipids in the Japanese. *Atherosclerosis* 100: 249-255.

McMurry, MP, MT Cerqueira, SL Connor, and WE Connor. 1991. Changes in lipid and lipoprotein levels and body weight in Tarahumara Indians after consumption of an affluent diet. *New Engl J Med* 325:1704-1708.

O'Dea, K. 1992. Obesity and diabetes in "the land of milk and honey." *Diabetes/Metab Rev* 8: 373-388.

Ravussin, E, PH Bennett, ME Valencia, LO Schulz, and J Esparza. 1994. Effects of a traditional lifestyle on obesity in Pima Indians. *Diabetes Care* 17: 1067-1074.

One Recipe, Two Results:
Insulin Resistance and Bad Body Fat

Anderson, JW, EC Konz, and DJ Jenkins. 2000. Health advantages and disadvantages of weight-reducing diets: a computer analysis and critical review. *J Am Coll Nutr* 19: 578-590.

Barnard, RJ, et al (cited in Chapters 3 and 6).

Cusin, I, F Rohner-Jeanrenaud, J Terrettaz, and B Jeanrenaud. 1992.

Hyperinsulinemia and its impact on obesity and insulin resistance. *Int J Obesity* 16 (Sup pl 4): S1-S11.

Hu, FB, JE Manson, MJ Stampfer, et al. 2001. Diet, lifestyle, and the risk of type 2 diabetes mellitus in women. *New Engl J Med* 345: 790-797.

Lemieux, S, and J-P Despres. 1994. Metabolic complications of visceral obesity: contribution to the aetiology of type 2 diabetes and implications for prevention and treatment. *Diabete & Metab (Paris)* 20: 375-393.

Randeree, HA, MAK Omar, AA Motala, and MA Seedat. 1992. Effect of insulin therapy on blood pressure in NIDDM patients with secondary failure. *Diabetes Care* 15: 1258-1263.

Sigal, RJ, M El-Hashimy, BC Martin, JS Soeldner, AS Krowlewski, and JH Warram. 1997. Acute postchallenge hyperinsulinemia predicts weight gain: a prospective study. *Diabetes* 46: 1025-1029.

van Dam, RM, EB Rimm, WC Willett, MJ Stampfer, and FB Hu. 2002. Dietary patterns and risk for type 2 diabetes mellitus in US men. *Ann Int Med* 136: 201-209.

The Twenty/Twenty Program for Metabolic Fitness

American Heart Association Nutrition Committee (A Chait, chair). 1993. Rationale of the Diet-Heart Statement of the American Heart Association. *Circulation* 88: 3008-3029.

Eaton, SB, M Shostak, and M Konner. 1988. *The Paleolithic Prescription: A Program of Diet and Exercise and a Design for Living*. New York: Harper & Row.

Weisburger, JH, and EL Wynder. 1991. Dietary fat intake and cancer. *Nutrition and Cancer* 5: 7-23.

Chapter Nine

Blair, SN, AL Dunn, BH Marcus, KH Cooper, and P Jaret. 2001. *Active Living Every Day: 20 Weeks To Lifelong Vitality*. Champaign, IL: Human Kinetics.

"Exercise Lite" for Metabolic Fitness

Pate, RR, et al. 1995. Physical activity and public health: a recommendation from the Centers for Disease Control and Prevention and the American College of Sports Medicine. *JAMA* 273: 402-407.

Stofan, JR, L DiPietro, D Davis, HW Kohl III, and SN Blair. 1998. Physical activity patterns associated with cardiorespiratory fitness and reduced mortality: the Aerobics Center Longitudinal Study. *Am J Pub Health* 88: 1807-1813.

Metabolic Fitness *versus* Cardiorespiratory Fitness:
Being Active *versus* Being "Fit"

Blair, SN, Y Cheng, and JS Holder. 2001. Is physical activity of physical fitness more important in defining health benefits? *Med Sci Sports Exerc* 33 (Suppl): S379-S399.

Blair, SN, et al. 1989. Idem. *JAMA* 262: 2395-2401.

Ekelund, L-G, WL Haskell, JL Johnson, FS Whaley, MH Criqui, and DS Sheps. 1988. Physical fitness as a predictor of cardiovascular mortality in asymptomatic North American men: the Lipid Research Clinic's mortality follow-up study. *N Engl J Med* 319: 1379-1384.

BIG FAT LIES

Hein, HO, P Suadicani, and F Gyntelberg. 1992. Physical fitness or physical activity as a predictor of ischaemic heart disease? A 17-year follow-up in the Copenhagen Male Study. *J Int Med* 232: 471-479.

Leon, AS, J Connett, DR Jacobs, and R Raurama. 1987. Leisure-time physical activity and risk of coronary heart disease and death: the Multiple Risk Factor Intervention Trial. *JAMA* 258: 2388-2395.

Sandvik, L, J Erikssen, E Thaulow, G Erikssen, R Mundal, and K Rodahl. 1993. Physical fitness as a predictor of mortality among healthy, middle-aged Norwegian men. *N Engl J Med* 328: 533-537.

The No-Sweat Way to Metabolic Fitness

Cononie, CC, AP Goldberg, E Rogus, and JM Hagberg. 1994. Seven consecutive days of exercise lowers plasma insulin responses to an oral glucose challenge in sedentary elderly. *J Am Geriatr Soc* 42: 394-398.

Despres, J-P, and B LaMarche. 1994. Low-intensity endurance exercise training, plasma lipoproteins and the risk of coronary heart disease. *J Int Med* 236: 7-22.

Despres, J-P. Obesity, regional adipose tissue distribution, and metabolism: effect of exercise. In: DR Romsos, et al, eds. 1991. *Obesity: Dietary Factors and Control.* Tokyo: Japan Sci. Soc. Press, pp. 251-259.

Hickey, MS, KE Gavigan, MR McCammon, et al. 1999. Effects of 7 days of exercise training on insulin action in morbidly obese men. *Clin Exer Physiol* 1: 24-28.

Oshida, Y, K Yamanouchi, S Hayamizu, and Y Sato. 1989. Long-term mild jogging increases insulin action despite no influence on body mass index or VO_2max. *J Appl Physiol* 66: 2206-2210.

Before You Start...

Astrand, P-O, and K Rodahl. 1970. *Textbook of Work Physiology.* New York: McGraw-Hill, p. 608.

Pratt, M. 1995. Exercise and sudden death: implications for health policy. *Sport Sci Rev* 4: 106-122.

Beyond the Two-Minute Walk

Boreham, CAG, WFM Wallace, and A Nevill. 2000. Training effects of accumulated daily stair-climbing exercise in previously sedentary young women. *Prev Med* 30: 277-281.

Coleman KJ, Raynor HR, Mueller DM, et al. 1999. Providing sedentary adults with choices for meeting their walking goals. *Prev Med* 28: 510-519.

Hu, FB, RJ Sigal, JW Rich-Edwards, et al. 1999. Walking compared with vigorous physical activity and risk of type 2 diabetes in women. *JAMA* 282: 1433-1439.

Jakicic JM, RR Wing, BA Butler, and RJ Robertson. 1995. Prescribing exercise in multiple short bouts *versus* one continuous bout: effects on adherence, cardiorespiratory fitness, and weight loss in overweight women. *Int J Obes* 19: 893-901.

Jakicic JM, C Winters, W Lang, and RR Wing. 1999. Effects of intermittent exercise and use of home exercise equipment on adherence, weight loss, and fitness in overweight women. *JAMA* 282: 1554-1560.

Lee, I-M, KM Rexrode, NR Cook, JE Manson, and JE Buring. 2001. Physical activity and coronary heart disease in women. Is "No pain, no gain" passé? *JAMA* 285: 1447-1454.

Lee I-M, HD Sesso, and RS Paffenbarger. 2000. Physical activity and coronary heart disease risk in men: Does the duration of exercise episodes predict risk? *Circulation* 102: 981-986.

Mensink, GBM, T Ziese, and FJ Kok. 1999. Benefits of leisure-time physical activity on the cardiovascular risk profile at older age. *Int J Epidemiol* 28: 659-666.

Murphy MH, and SE Hardman. 1998. Training effects of short and long bouts of brisk walking in sedentary women. *Med Sci Sports Exerc* 30: 152-157.

Parkkari, J, A Natri, P Kannus, et al. 2000. A controlled trial of the health benefits of regular walking on a golf course. *Am J Med* 109: 102-108.

No Pain, Lots of Gain: Regulating Intensity

American College of Sports Medicine. 1993. Position Stand: Physical activity, physical fitness, and hypertension. *Med Sci Sports Exerc* 25: i-x.

Belman, MJ, and GA Gaesser. 1991. Exercise training below and above the lactate threshold in the elderly. *Med Sci Sports Exerc* 232: 562-568.

Borg, G. 1982. Psychophysical bases of perceived exertion. *Med Sci Sports Exerc* 14: 377-381.

Borg, G. 1990. Psychophysical scaling with applications in physical work and the perception of exertion. *Scand J Work Environ Health* 16 (Suppl 1): 55-58.

Duncan, JJ, NF Gordon, and CB Scott. 1991. Women walking for health and fitness: how much is enough? *JAMA* 266: 3295-3299.

Gaesser, GA, and RG Rich. 1984. Effects of high- and low-intensity exercise training on aerobic capacity and blood lipids. *Med Sci Sports Exerc* 16: 269-274.

Spelman, CC, RR Pate, CA Macera, and DS Ward. 1993. Self-selected exercise intensity of habitual walkers. *Med Sci Sports Exerc* 25: 1174-1179.

Warming Up, Cooling Down, and Stretching

Nelson, ME, MA Fiatarone, CM Morganti, I Trice, RA Greenberg, and WJ Evans. 1994. Effects of high-intensity strength training on multiple risk factors for osteoporotic fractures. *JAMA* 272: 1909-1914.

It's Never Too Late to Start

Blair, SN, HW Kohl III, CE Barlow, RS Paffenbarger, LW Gibbons, and CA Macera. 1995. Changes in physical fitness and all-cause mortality: a prospective study of healthy and unhealthy men. *JAMA* 273: 1093-1098.

Erikssen, G, K Liestol, J Bjorntorp, E Thaulow, L Sandvik, and J Eriksson. 1998. Changes in physical fitness and changes in mortality. *Lancet* 352: 759-762.

Paffenbarger, RS, RT Hyde, AL Wing, I-M Lee, DL Jung, and JB Kampert. 1993. The association of changes in physical-activity level and other lifestyle characteristics with mortality among men. *N Engl J Med* 328: 538-545.

Wannamethee, SG, AG Shaper, and M Walker. 1998. Changes in physical activity, mortality, and incidence of coronary heart disease in older men. *Lancet* 351: 1603-1608.

Chapter Ten

Begley, S (with K Springen and M Hager). April 25, 1994. Beyond vitamins. *Newsweek*, pp. 45-49.

Pritikin, N. Sept./Oct. 1984. Food poisoning: a major health problem in the United States. *The Humanist*, pp. 5-9, 32.

Carbohydrates and Fats: Some Definitions

Ascherio, A, MB Katan, PL Zock, MJ Stampfer, and WC Willett. 1999. Trans fatty acids and coronary heart disease. *New Engl J Med* 340: 1994-1998.

Dolnick, E. Oct. 1992. Beyond the French Paradox. *Health*, pp. 40-49.

Kromhout, D, EB Bosschieter, and C de Lezenne Coulander. 1985. The inverse relation between fish consumption and 20-year mortality from coronary heart disease. *N Engl J Med* 312: 1205-1209.

Mann, GV. Metabolic consequences of dietary trans fatty acids. *Lancet* 343: 1268-1271, 1994.

Univ. of California at Berkeley Wellness Letter, Oct. 1994, p. 3.

Univ. of California at Berkeley Wellness Letter, Sept. 1993, pp. 4-6.

Starting the Nutritional Component of the Twenty/Twenty Program: The High-Carbohydrate Way to Health

Anderson, JW. 2000. Dietary fiber prevents carbohydrate-induced hypertriglyceridemia. *Cur Atherosc Rep* 2: 536-541.

Blackburn, GL. 1992. Improving the American diet. *Am J Public Health* 82: 465-466.

Block G (quoted in: R Schoch) June 1994. Vitamins are good medicine. *California Monthly*, pp. 18-19.

Jenkins, DJ, CW Kendall, DG Popovich, et al. 2001. Effect of a very-high-fiber vegetable, fruit, and nut diet on seum lipids and colonic function. *Metab: Clin Exp* 50: 494-503.

Kennedy, ET, SA Bowman, JT Spence, M Freedman, and J King. 2001. Popular diets: correlation to health, nutrition, and obesity. *J Am Diet Assoc* 101: 411-420.

Khaw, K-T, and E Barrett-Connor. 1987. Dietary fiber and reduced ischemic heart disease mortality rates in men and women: A 12-year prospective study. *Am J Epidemiol* 126: 1093-1102.

Kritchevsky, D. The role of fat, calories, and fiber in disease. In: FN Kotsonis, M Mackey, and J Hjelle, eds. 1994. *Nutritional Toxicology*, New York: Raven Press, pp. 67-93.

Liu, S, JE Buring, HD Sesso, EB Rimm, WC Willett, and JE Manson. 2002. A prospective study of dietary fiber intake and risk of cardiovascular disease among women. *J Am Coll Cardiol* 39: 49-56.

Patterson, BH, G Block, WF Rosenberger, D Pees, and LL Kahls. 1990. Fruits and vegetables in the American diet: data from the NHANES II survey. *Am J Public Health* 80: 1443-1449.

Rimm, EB, A Ascherio, E Giovannucci, D Spiegelman, MJ Stampfer, and WC Willett. 1996. Vegetable, fruit, and cereal fiber intake and risk of coronary heart disease among men. *JAMA* 275: 447-451.

Van Horn, L, A Moag-Stahlberg, K Liu, C Ballew, K Ruth, R Hughes, and J Stamler. 1991. Effects on serum lipids of adding instant oats to usual American diets. *Am J Public Health* 81: 183-188.

Willett, WC. 1994. Diet and health: what should we eat? *Science* 264: 532-537.

Wolever, TMS. 1991. Diet and blood lipid levels: effect of "nibbling." *Can Med Assoc J* 144: 729.

Wolk, A, JE Manson, MJ Stampfer, et al. 1999. Long-term intake of dietary fiber and decreased risk of coronary heart disease among women. *JAMA* 281: 1998-2004.

Eating More Complex Carbohydrates
Won't Make You Gain Weight

Acheson, KJ. 1993. Do carbohydrates make you fat? *Nutrition* 9: 185.

Acheson, KJ, Y Schutz, T Bessard, E Ravussin, E Jequier, and JP Flatt. 1984. Nutritional influences on lipogenesis and thermogenesis after a carbohydrate meal. *Am J Physiol 246* (*Endocrinol Metab* 9): E62-E70.

Danforth, E. 1985. Diet and obesity. *Am J Clin Nutr* 41: 1132-1145.

Kennedy, ET, et al. 2001. Idem. *J Am Diet Assoc* 101: 411-420.

Poppitt, SD, GF Keogh, AM Prentice, et al. 2002. Long-term effects of ad libitum low-fat, high-carbohydrate diets on body weight and serum lipids in overweight subjects with metabolic syndrome. *Am J Clin Nutr* 75: 11-20.

Prewitt, TE, D Schmeisser, PE Bowen, P Aye, TA Dolecek, P Langenberg, T Cole, and L Brace. 1991. Changes in body weight, body composition, and energy intake in women fed high- and low-fat diets. *Am J Clin Nutr* 54: 304-310.

How To Figure out
How Many Grams of Fat Equal 20 Percent

Ehnholm, C, et al. 1982. Idem. *N Engl J Med* 307: 850-855.

Getting to 20 Percent Fat
with the Help of the USDA Food Pyramid

Kant, AK, A Schatzkin, TB Harris, RG Ziegler, and G Block. 1993. Dietary diversity and subsequent mortality in the first National Health and Nutrition Examination Survey Epidemiologic follow-up study. *Am J Clin Nutr* 57: 434-440.

US Department of Agriculture, Human Nutrition Information Service. *Dietary Guidelines and Your Diet. Home and Garden Bulletin*, No. 232-1 through 232-11.

USDA. 1998. USDA continuing survey of food intakes by individuals, 1994-1996.

Metabolic Fitness in a Pill?

Campfield, LA, FJ Smith, Y Guisez, R Devos, and P Burn. 1995. Recombinant mouse OB protein: evidence for a peripheral signal linking adiposity and central neural networks. *Science* 269: 546-549.

Diabetes Prevention Program Research Group. 2002. Reduction in the incidence of type 2 diabetes with lifestyle intervention or metformin. *New Engl J Med* 346: 393-403.

Halaas, JL, KS Gajiwala, M Maffei, et al. 1995. Weight-reducing effects of the plasma protein encoded by the obese gene. *Science* 269: 543-546.

Hamilton, BS, D Paglia, AYM Kwan, and M Deitel. 1995. Increased obese mRNA expression in omental fat cells from massively obese humans. *Nature Med* 1: 953-956.

Heymsfield, SB, AS Greenberg, K Fujioka, et al. 1999. Recombinant leptin for weight loss in obese and lean adults. *JAMA* 282: 1568-1575.

Lonnqvist, F, P Arner, L Nordfors, and M Schalling. 1995. Overexpression of the obese (ob) gene in adipose tissue of human obese subjects. *Nature Med* 1: 950-953.

Zhang, Y, R Proenca, M Maffei, M Barone, L Leopold, and JM Friedman. 1994. Positional cloning of the mouse obese gene and its human homologue. *Nature* 372: 425-432.

RECOMMENDED READING

Berg, Frances. *Children and Teens Afraid to Eat: Helping Youth in Today's Weight-Obsessed World.* Hettinger, North Dakota: Healthy Weight Publishing Network, 1999.

Berg, Frances. *Women Afraid To Eat: Breaking Free in Today's Weight-Obsessed World.* Hettinger, North Dakota: Healthy Weight Publishing Network, 2000.

Bernell, Bonnie. *Bountiful Women: Large Women's Secrets for Living the Life They Desire.* Berkeley, CA: Wildcat Canyon Press, 2000.

Bevere, Lisa. *You Are Not What You Weigh: Escaping the Lie and Living the Truth.* Orlando, FL: Creation House, 1999.

Bevere, Lisa. *The True Measure of a Woman: You Are More than What You See.* Orlando, FL: Creation House, 1997.

Bliss, Kelly. *Don't Weight: Get Moving and Eat Healthy Now.* Philadelphia, PA: Xlibris Corporation, 2001.

Boston Women's Health Collective. *Our Bodies, Ourselves for the New Century: A Book by and for Women.* New York: Touchstone Books, 1998.

Bruno, Barbara Altman. *Worth Your Weight: What You Can Do about a Weight Problem.* Bethel, CT: Rutledge Books, 1996.

Chernin, Kim. *The Obsession: Reflections on the Tyranny of Slenderness.* New York: Harper & Row, 1981.

Chernin, Kim. *The Hungry Self: Women, Eating and Identity.* New York: Harper & Row, 1985.

Colles, Lisa, and Andrew Prentice. *Fat: Exploding the Myths.* New York: Welcome Rain, 1999.

Cooke, Kaz. *Real Gorgeous: The Truth about Body and Beauty.* New York: WW Norton and Company, 1998.

Cordes, Helen. *Girl Power in the Mirror: A Book about Girls, Their Bodies, and Themselves.* Minneapolis, MN: Lerner Publications Company, 2000.

Edut, Ophira. *Body Outlaws: Young Women Write about Body Image and Identity*. Seattle: Seal Press, 2000.

Erdman, Cheri K. *Nothing to Lose: A Guide to Sane Living in a Larger Body*. San Francisco: Harper SanFrancisco, 1995.

Fraser, Laura. *Losing It: False Hopes and Fat Profits in the Diet Industry*. New York: Plume, 1998.

Freedman, Rita. *Bodylove: Learning to Like Our Looks and Ourselves*. Carlsbad, CA: Gürze Books, 2002.

Friedman, Sandra Susan. *When Girls Feel Fat—Helping Girls through Adolescence*. Buffalo, NY: Firefly Books, 2000.

Gaesser, Glenn, and Karin Kratina. *Eating Well, Living Well: When You Can't Diet Anymore*. Parker, CO: Wheat Foods Council, 2000.

Garrison, Terry. *Fed-up! A Woman's Guide to Liberation from the Diet/Weight Prison*. New York: Carroll & Graf, 1993.

Goodman, W. Charisse. *The Invisible Woman: Confronting Weight Prejudice in America*. Carlsbad, CA: Gürze Books, 1995.

Hakala, Dee. *Thin Is Just a Four-letter Word*. New York: Dell, 1997.

Hillman, Carolynn. *Love Your Looks: How to Stop Criticizing and Start Appreciating Your Appearance*. New York: Simon & Schuster, 1996.

Hirschmann, Jane R., and Carol H. Munter. *Overcoming Overeating*. New York: Fawcett Columbine, 1988.

Hirschmann, Jane R., and Carol H. Munter. *When Women Stop Hating Their Bodies: Freeing Yourself from Food and Weight Obsession*. New York: Fawcett Columbine, 1995.

Hutchison, Marcia. *Transforming Body Image: Learning to Love the Body You Have*. Freedom, CA: Crossing Press, 1985.

Ikeda, Joanne, and Priscilla Naworski. *Am I Fat? Helping Your Children Accept Differences in Body Size*. Santa Cruz, California: ETR Associates, 1992.

Johnson, Carol. *Self-Esteem Comes in All Sizes: How to be Happy and Healthy at Your Natural Weight*. Carlsbad, CA: Gürze Books, 2001.

Jonas, Steven, and Linda Konner. *Just the Weigh You Are: How to be Fit and Healthy, Whatever Your Size*. Shelburne, VT: Chapters Publishing, 1997.

Kilbourne, Jean. *Can't Buy My Love: How Advertising Changes the Way We Think and Feel.* New York: Touchstone Books, 1999.

Kratina, Karin, Nancy L. King, and Dayle Hayes. *Moving Away From Diets: New Ways to Heal Eating Problems & Exercise Resistance.* Lake Dallas, TX: Helm Seminars, 1996.

Lyons, Pat, and Debby Burgard. *Great Shape: The First Fitness Guide for Large Women.* Lincoln, NJ: iUniverse.com, 2000.

MacKoff, Barbara. *Growing a Girl: Seven Strategies for Raising a Strong, Spirited Daughter.* New York: Dell Publishing, 1996.

Manheim, Camryn. *Wake Up, I'm Fat!* New York: Broadway Books, 1999.

Mayer, Ken. *Real Women Don't Diet! One Man's Praise of Large Women and His Outrage at the Society That Rejects Them.* Silver Spring, MD: Bartleby Press, 1993.

The Melpomene Institute for Women's Research. *The Bodywise Woman.* New York: Prentice-Hall, 1992.

Mundy, Alicia. *Dispensing with the Truth: The Victims, the Drug Companies, and the Dramatic Story Behind the Battle over Fen-Phen.* New York: St. Martin's Press, 2001.

Newman, Lesléa. *SomeBody to Love.* Chicago: Third Side Press, 1991.

Newman, Lesléa. *Fat Chance.* New York: The Putnam & Grosset Group, 1994.

Northrup, Christine. *Women's Bodies, Women's Wisdom: Creating Physical and Emotional Health and Healing.* New York: Bantam, 1994.

O'Garden, Irene. *Fat Girl: One Woman's Way Out.* San Francisco: Harper SanFrancisco, 1993.

Omichinski, Linda. *You Count, Calories Don't.* Manitoba, Canada: Hyperion, 1992.

Omichinski, Linda. *Staying Off the Diet Roller Coaster.* Washington, DC: Advice Zone, 2000.

Poulton, Terry. *No Fat Chicks. How Women Are Brainwashed to Hate Their Bodies and Spend Their Money.* Toronto: Key Porter Books, 1996.

Rice, Rochelle. *Real Fitness for Real Women: A Unique Workout Program for the Plus-Size Woman.* New York: Warner Books, 2001.

Roberts, Nancy. *Breaking All the Rules: Feeling Good and Looking Great No Matter What Your Size.* New York: Penguin Books, 1985.

Rodin, Judith. *Body Traps.* New York: Quill William Morrow, 1992.

Rose, Laura. *Life Isn't Weighed on the Bathroom Scale.* Waco, TX: WRS Publishing, 1993.

Satter, Ellyn. *How to Get Your Kids to Eat...But Not Too Much—From Birth to Adolescence.* Palo Alto, CA: Bull Publishing Company, 1987.

Satter, Ellyn. *Child of Mine—Feeding with Love and Good Sense.* Palo Alto, CA: Bull Publishing Company, 2000.

Satter, Ellyn. *Secrets of Feeding a Healthy Family.* Madison, WI: Kelcy Press, 1999.

Schwartz, Hillel. *Never Satisfied: A Cultural History of Diets, Fantasies and Fat.* New York: The Free Press, 1986.

Sobal, Jeffery, and Donna Maurer. *Interpreting Weight: The Social Management of Fatness and Thinness.* New York: Aldine de Gruyter, 1999.

Sobal, Jeffery, and Donna Maurer. *Weight Issues: Fatness and Thinness as Social Problems.* New York: Aldine de Gruyter, 1999.

Solovay, Sondra. *Tipping the Scales of Justice: Fighting Weight-Based Discrimination.* Amherst, NY: Prometheus Books, 2000.

Sullivan, Judy. *Size Wise: A Catalog of More than 1000 Resources for Living with Confidence and Comfort at Any Size.* New York: Avon, 1997.

Thompson, J. Kevin; Leslie J. Heinberg; Madeline Altabe; and Stacey Tantleff-Dunn. *Exacting Beauty: Theory, Assessment, and Treatment of Body Image Disturbance.* Washington, DC: American Psychological Association, 1999.

Vandereycken, Walter, and Greta Noordenbos. *Studies in Eating Disorders—An International Series: The Prevention of Eating Disorders.* London: The Athlone Press, 1998.

Wann, Marilyn. *Fat!So? Because You Don't Have to Apologize for Your Size.* Berkeley, CA: Ten Speed Press, 1999.

Wiley, Carol. *Journeys to Self-Acceptance: Fat Women Speak.* Freedom, CA: The Crossing Press, 1998.

Wolf, Naomi. *The Beauty Myth: How Images of Beauty Are Used against Women.* New York: William Morrow, 1991.

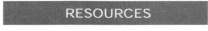

Organizations, Magazines, and Websites that Promote Health at Every Size

About Face
Positive self-esteem in girls and women
P. O. Box 77665
San Francisco, CA 94107
(415) 436-0212
info@about-face.org
www.about-face.org

Abundia Retreats
Weekend retreats for the larger woman
Contact person: Barbara Spaulding
(847) 705-9256

Amplestuff
P.O. Box 116
Bearsville, NY 12409-0116
amplestuff@aol.com
www.amplestuff.com

ANAD (National Assoc. of Anorexia Nervosa and Associated Disorders)
P.O. Box 7
Highland Park, IL 60035
(708) 831-3438
www.anad.org

Beyond Bias Diversity Training
(510) 839-8743

Sondra@BeyondBias.com
www.BeyondBias.com

Big As Texas
P.O. Box 363
Sour Lake, TX 77659
(409) 753-3451
BigAsTexas@juno.com
www.members.tripod.com/bigastexas

Big Beautiful Woman Magazine Online
www.bbwmagazine.com

Big Folks Exercise and Fitness Resources FAQ (Frequently Asked Questions)
www.faqs.org/faqs/fat-acceptance-faq/fitness

Fitness & Healthy Living with Bliss™
www.kellybliss.com

Body Image Task Force (BITF)
P.O. Box 360196
Melbourne, FL 32936-0196
bitf@yahoo.com
www.home.earthlink.net/~dawn_atkins/bitf.htm

Body Positive
Boosting body image at any weight
www.bodypositive.com

The Body Positive
1115 Evelyn Ave.
Albany, CA 94706
(510) 841-9389
www.thebodypositive.org

CASA (Canadian Association for Size Acceptance)
Suite 511 - 99 Dalhousie Street
Toronto, Ontario M5B 2N2
(416) 861-0217

cdawyde@interlog.com
www.interlog.com/~cdawyde

Center for Weight and Health at U.C. Berkeley
www.cnr.berkeley.edu/cwh

Council on Size and Weight Discrimination
P.O. Box 305
Mt. Marion, NY 12456
Miriam@cswd.org
www.cswd.org

Dads and Daughters
www.dadsanddaughters.org

Eating Disorder Referral and Information Center
2923 Sandy Pointe, Suite 6
Del Mar, CA 92014-2052
(858) 481-1515
Fax: (858) 481-5143
www.edreferral.com

Feeling Good Fitness
Contact person: Jennifer Portnick
www.feelinggoodfitness.com

Food and Nutrition Information Center
National clearinghouse on nutrition information and resource list on
eating disorders
www.nal.usda.gov/fnic/pubs_and_db.html
www.nal.usda.gov/fnic/pubs/bibs/gen/eatingdis.htm

Girl Power!
Sponsored by U.S. Dept. of Health and Human Services
www.girlpower.gov

Girl Zone
www.girlzone.com

Gürze Books
P.O. Box 2238
Carlsbad, CA
(800) 756-7533
www.bulimia.com

Healthy Weight Network
402 South 14th Street
Hettinger, ND 58639
(701) 567-2646
Fax: (701) 567-2602
www.healthyweightnetwork.com

Holistic Health Promotion/Health at Every Size
Contact person: Jonathan Isaac Robison Ph.D., M.S.
www.jonrobison.net

HUGS International
Box 102 A, RR #3
Portage la Prairie, Manitoa R1N 3A3
(204) 428-3432
Fax: (204) 428-5072
linda@hugs.com
www.hugs.com

ISAA (International Size-Acceptance Association)
P.O. Box 82126
Austin, TX 78758
Director@size-acceptance.org
www.size-acceptance.org

Largely Positive, Inc.
Carol Johnson, Director
P.O. Box 170223
Glendale, WI 53217
(414) 299-9295 (voicemail)
positive@execpc.com
www.largelypositive.com

Largesse, the Network for Size Esteem
Fax: (707) 929-1612
largesse@eskimo.com
www.eskimo.com/~largesse

Melpomene Institute for Women's Health Research
1010 University Avenue
St. Paul, MN 55104
(651) 642-1951
Fax: (651) 642-1871
health@melpomene.org
www.melpomene.org

NAAFA (National Association to Advance Fat Acceptance)
P.O. Box 188620
Sacramento, CA 95818
(916) 558-6880
naafa@naafa.org
www.naafa.org

National Eating Disorders Association
603 Stewart St., Suite 803
Seattle, WA 98101
(206) 382-3587
www.nationaleatingdisorders.org

NEDIC (National Eating Disorders Centre)
CW1-211/200 Elizabeth Street
Toronto, Ontario M5G 2C4
Program Coordinator: Karin Davis
(416) 340-4800 ext. 8114
karin.davis@uhn.on.ca
www.nedic.ca

New Moon
Nurturing the development of strong, confident girls
www.newmoon.org

Overcoming Overeating
www.overcomingovereating.com

Radiance Magazine Online
www.radiancemagazine.com

The Renfrew Center Foundation
475 Spring Lane
Philadelphia, PA 19128
www.renfrew.org

Sandie's Clothesline
Contact person: Sandie Sabo
P.O. Box 130244
Carlsbad, CA 92013
(760) 918-0909

Size Wise
www.sizewise.com

Venus Group
A social and support network for large women
P.O. Box 8126
Ann Arbor, MI 48107
(734) 327-4936
hmacallister@hotmail.com

Weight-control Information Network (WIN)
www.niddk.nih.gov/health/nutrit/win.htm
(for "Active at Any Size" pamphlet:
www.niddk.nih.gov/health/nutrit/activeatanysize/active.html#activeat)

Y

Glenn A. Gaesser, Ph.D.

Glenn Gaesser, Ph.D., is a professor of exercise physiology and director of the Kinesiology Program at the University of Virginia. A Phi Beta Kappa graduate from the University of California at Berkeley and a Fellow of the American College of Sports Medicine, Dr. Gaesser has conducted research and published many articles on exercise, health, and fitness in scientific journals, trade publications, and newsletters, and has presented frequently at national and international meetings on the subject of body weight and health.

He has appeared on Good Morning America, ABC's 20/20, World News Tonight with Peter Jennings, NBC Nightly News, CNN, and Dateline NBC. In addition, he has been a guest on dozens of radio shows in North America and has been interviewed for stories on body weight, fitness, and health for numerous newspapers and magazines.

He lives with his wife and children in Charlottesville, Virginia.

BIG FAT LIES is available at bookstores and libraries or may be ordered directly from Gürze Books.

FREE Catalogue

The Eating Disorders Resource Catalogue has more than 200 books on eating disorders and related topics, including body image, size-acceptance, self-esteem, and more. It is a valuable resource that includes listings of non-profit associations and treatment facilities, and it is handed out by therapists, educators, and other health care professionals throughout the world. Additional resources are also available at *www.bulimia.com*.

Please indicate quantity:

___ FREE copies of the *Eating Disorders Resource Catalogue*.

___ copies of *BIG FAT LIES*
    $15.95 per copy plus $3.00 each for shipping.
    Quantity discounts are available.

Name _____

Address _____

City, St, Zip _____

Phone _____

Gürze Books
P.O. Box 2238
Carlsbad, CA 92018
(800) 756-7533
www.gurze.com